Making Health Decisions

Thomas M. Vogt

Making Health Decisions

An Epidemiologic Perspective on Staying Well

Nelson-Hall **nh** Chicago

53965

RA
651
V6
1983

#*94/2968*

LIBRARY OF CONGRESS CATALOGING IN PUBLICATION DATA

Vogt, Thomas M.
   Making health decisions.

   Includes bibliographical references and index.
   1. Epidemiology.   2. Health.   3. Health behavior.
4. Medicine, Preventive.   I. Title.   [DNLM:
1. Epidemiology—Popular works.   2. Health.   WA 105
V887m]
RA651.V6   1983   614.4   83-6260
ISBN 0-8304-1001-5

Manufactured in the United States of America

10 9 8 7 6 5 4 3 2 1

The paper in this book is pH neutral (acid-free).

*To David L. Jameson and
S. Leonard Syme, both living
illustrations of the adage that
a good teacher is worth a
thousand books.*

Contents

Preface

For several years now a part of my income has been derived from helping persons with high risk of illness to reduce that risk by adopting more healthy behaviors and practices. In that time I have become something of an expert on what I call the "everything-is-bad-for-you-anyhow" syndrome. This often serious malady is a product of several causes working in concert. These include a bit of cynicism, a dash of rationalization, and a large dollop of the popular press.

Those of us who dwell at least part of the time in the ivory tower of research tend to forget that there is a large industry out there interpreting the results of our research for the general public. This amnesia may well be the scientist's version of the old head-in-the-sand response so favored by metaphorical ostriches. Invariably, a review of health information available to the general public reveals an appalling lack of balance. The result is a populace besieged by claims, often conflicting, that various nostrums, practices, diets, vapors, chemicals, and other assorted items will kill and/or cure. One major national tabloid seems compelled to discover a cure for cancer at least once every two or three weeks and a cure for heart disease about once every six weeks. Presumably cancer sells better than heart disease, even though the latter kills nearly four times as often. As a consequence, it is hardly surprising that both the public and physicians are confused about what things are risky and what things are not. This is frequently translated to the "everything-is-bad-for-you-anyhow" syndrome in which complete skepticism and inaction reign.

This book is designed to help the reader plot a reasonable course through this turbulent sea of claims and counterclaims. The results of population-based epidemiological research over the past thirty years have consistently and clearly identified a few very important factors which substantially increase our risk of disease and death. In addition, other factors have been noted which may be harmful (or helpful), but for which sufficient evidence is not yet available to warrant changes in our lives or practices. Finally, many false claims have been laid to rest. Old wives have been detected among some of the old tales. It is not the purpose of this book to provide any comprehensive listing of what is good for you and what is not. Such a list would inevitably be obsolete within a few years. Several health risks will, however, be discussed as examples.

It is my hope to provide the tools with which the reader can make judgments about the information he or she reads with respect to health and disease. These tools are not overly complex and ought to be taught to all of us while we are in school. The book is not heavily referenced. Too many references distract from the flow of reading and also allow authors to hide behind the opinions of others. Enough references are provided to enable any reader, sufficiently motivated, to begin a search of the relevant scientific literature. Most of those cited sources have substantial bibliographies of their own.

A second reason that this book rests in your hands relates to the author's frustration at always being mistaken for a skin doctor. Epidemiology, as will be repeated again and again, has absolutely nothing to do with skin diseases. It is, rather, a simple, straightforward method for determining (or at least making educated guesses about) cause and effect by examining large groups of people instead of individuals. Despite the fact that this discipline is very little known, it has already profoundly affected your life, as you will see, and its basic approaches to understanding health and disease can be your own tools for evaluating the relative strengths and weaknesses of the health-related claims you read in your daily paper. The lack of published material dealing with this issue seems surprising in view of our society's increasing concerns over personal responsibility for health. I hope that this first attempt will stimulate further and better efforts in the same direction.

The author gratefully acknowledges the editorial assistance of Margaret Sucec, the clerical work of Sharon Patterson, Debbie Schoenheinz, Karen Stokes, and Phyllis Snedeker, and the encouragement and inspiration of M. R. Greenlick.

Chapter 1
What Epidemiology Is

Why This Book Will Not Cure Your Skin Problems

If you believe everything, you are not a believer in anything at all.

—*Idries Shah*

It is more than a little frustrating to belong to a profession that nine out of ten people do not recognize, and all the more so because it is invariably mistaken for another which is completely unrelated to it. Cocktail parties can become nightmares. Following an introduction, the conversation often runs like this:

"And what are you?"

"I beg your pardon?"

"Your work. What kind of work do you do?"

"Oh, I'm an epidemiologist."

"That's fascinating. You know, I have this problem with zits on my chin that just keep coming. What can I do about it?"

"I really wouldn't know. Epidemiology has nothing to do with the skin. It's the study of health and illness in large groups of people in order to determine their causes and prevention. It . . . now, where did she get off to?"

This confusion about the nature of epidemiology is amplified by the fact that epidemiologists themselves cannot agree on what it is they do. So much controversy has been generated within the field that in 1978 the *American Journal of Epidemiology* carried an article entitled "Definitions of Epidemiology" (see table 1.1), in which the author cited twenty-three definitions from the literature, then felt compelled to offer his own.[1] Several months later a reply in the letters-to-the-editor column offered still another definition. None of these, however, are my own favorite definition: Epidemiology is what epidemiologists do.

Following the often misguided apprehension that it is informative to examine the etymological origins of a word, the word *epidemiology* has three Greek roots: *epi* (upon), *demos* (people), and *logos* (study of). Thus, it might be defined as the "study of what is upon the people." That doesn't help much.

Epidemiology has grown from the concern of physicians during the last two centuries with the prevention of illness and the desire to understand its causes. Traditionally, a physician examines a patient, and by putting together clues arising from the patient's condition, he or she can arrive at a kind of gestalt which allows a diagnosis to be made. Usually, there are pieces of the physical picture which don't quite fit, but, taking everything else into account, such anomalies will not often mislead the healer. Given a diagnosis, the physician has been trained also in the treatment of that condition, and, consequently, will then do the best he or she can to effect a cure, or to support the patient in effecting the cure. The epidemiologist studies populations of people the way the physician studies individuals. By observing the patterns of occurrence of disease, the epidemiologist arrives at a gestalt—not of diagnosis, but of cause. The physician is primarily a diagnoser and healer. That is the orientation of medical school and the focus of medical technology.

Over the centuries healers of many sorts have been unsatisfied with this somewhat limited role. Clearly, it does not address the cause of the illness except as it relates to diagnosis and treatment. It does nothing to prevent a recurrence in the same person or in others. I spent the years 1964 to 1966 working with the Peace Corps in Ethiopia. At that time there was a fledgling medical school in Addis Ababa, the capital city, and quite a large number of hospitals as well. There was little medical care elsewhere in the country, but what there was consisted of small local clinics and regional hospitals. There was essentially no public health effort. Addis Ababa was reputed to be the largest city in the world lacking a sewage system. Water mains were buried next to open and contaminated streams. The ultimate irony was that this poor government was bearing the substantial costs of a medical school and large, acute-care hospitals while paying no attention to preventing disease. A man with dysentery might get treated at a clinic, return home, and catch dysentery again the next day. The money spent on such medical care was totally wasted, and it occurred to me that, perhaps, there is a measure of that waste in our own society as well.

LASSA FEVER—AN EPIDEMIOLOGIC INVESTIGATION

The techniques of epidemiology are easiest to illustrate with investigations into the sources of infectious illnesses. Public health departments around the world hire epidemiologists to identify unusual outbreaks of disease, investigate them, and locate and interrupt the sources of infection. A number of years ago New Yorker magazine carried a series entitled "Annals of Epidemiology" by Berton Roueche which related these investigations as if they were detective stories, as indeed they often are. These essays have been published as a popular collection and they provide entertaining reading.[2]

TABLE 1.1
Selected Summary of Definitions of Epidemiology

Date	Author	Definition
1927	Frost	"The science of the mass-phenomena of infectious diseases, or as the natural history of infectious diseases; . . . concerned not merely with describing the distribution of disease, but equally or more fitting it into a consistent philosophy"
1931	Stallybrass	"the science of the infective diseases—their prime causes, propagation and prevention"
1934	Greenwood	"the study of disease as a mass phenomenon"
1938	Paul	"concerned with circumstances . . . where disease is prone to develop"
1943	Aycock	"Epidemiology must understand disease, not so much as it affects the individual or as it behaves under the eye of the observer at any one time or in any one place, but as it imposes itself on groups of people even if they extend across boundaries set by men for economic, political, and social purposes. . . ."
1951	Maxcy	"that field of medical science which is concerned with the relationships of the various factors and conditions which determine the frequencies and distributions of an infectious process, a disease, or a physiological state in a human community"
1958	Stamler	"the study of disease in populations"
1958	Lilienfeld	"the study of the distribution of a disease or condition in a population of those factors which influence their distribution"
1961	Reid	"deals with the characteristic behaviour of such diseases within the complex matrix of human populations"

Year	Author	Definition
1962	Pemberton	"the study of the laws governing the distribution of disease in the community"
1963	Cockburn	"the study of the ecology of infectious diseases"
1963	Gordon	"the study of disease as it occurs in nature"
1967	Taylor	"the study of health or ill health in a defined population"
1970	Fox et al.	"the study of factors determining the occurrence of disease in populations"
1970	MacMahon & Pugh	"the study of the distribution and determinants of disease frequency in man"
1973	Sartwell	"the study of the distribution and dynamics of diseases in human populations"
1973	Lowe & Kostrzewski	"the study of the factors determining the frequency and distribution of disease in human populations"
1974	Mausner & Bahn	"the study of the distribution and determinants of diseases and injuries in human populations"
1974	Friedman	"the study of disease occurrence in human populations"
1975	Morris	"the basic science of preventive and community medicine"
1975	Lasagna	"the science dealing with the incidence, spread, and control of disease"
1976	Lilienfeld	"the study of the distribution of a disease or a physiological condition in human populations and of the factors that influence this distribution"
1976	Sinnecker	"concerned with mass outbreaks of disease"

SOURCE: Adapted from D. E. Lilienfeld, "Definitions of Epidemiology," *American Journal of Epidemiology* 107 (1978): 87–90.
Reprinted with permission of the author and publisher.

Perhaps the most dramatic epidemiologic investigation of recent years, though, was that which surrounded the outbreak of a new disease in Lassa, Nigeria.[3] In January of 1969, an elderly medical missionary named Laura Wine became ill with symptoms that were not readily identifiable by the hospital staff at her mission. She had fever, weakness, and a strange group of yellowish ulcers, which were surrounded by halos, at the back of her throat. She did not respond to penicillin or other medical therapy. Her kidneys failed, and she was flown with great difficulty to the city of Jos, high on the central Nigerian plateau. She developed heart failure at the hospital, but still no specific diagnosis could be made. Shortly thereafter she died. An autopsy revealed internal hemorrhaging, but all bacterial and viral cultures were negative.

Eight days later a second staff member became sick with similar symptoms. Eleven days later she also died. A week later a third nurse, Penny Pinneo, became ill. She was evacuated to the United States. The arbovirus laboratory at Yale University was given the task of searching for the cause of the mysterious malady that afflicted the gravely ill woman. The details of the investigation are too intricate to provide in any depth here, but even a brief outline is fascinating. Pinneo was taken to Columbia Presbyterian Hospital in New York City and placed under strict isolation. The fact that three co-workers had been afflicted with the same condition suggested that it was highly communicable. The deaths of two indicated that the condition did not respond to medical therapy and that the risks of exposure might be substantial. This risk applied also to those laboratory workers who had to handle the blood and urine specimens used for testing. Strict controls were essential. These specimens were injected into mice in hopes of growing the organism responsible for the disease. But the infant mice didn't get sick, while cells grown in cultures and exposed to infected materials were riddled with white virus-induced markings. That seemed strange, and it was originally thought that a contaminant might be responsible. Meanwhile, Penny Pinneo, who had already survived longer than either of the other two victims, was growing sicker. Her ears rang, her ability to hear declined, her blood failed to clot properly, and her heart and kidney functions deteriorated.

The repeat cultures proved that contamination had not been the cause of the original results. Why, then, did the infant mice not get sick? Perhaps, it was thought, because they did not react to the virus like older mice would. Adult mice were then injected for the first time and they rapidly sickened and died. But the clinical picture was strange, unexpectedly like a South American type of virus. As lower and lower doses of the virus were given to mice, it was apparent how extraordinarily powerful they were. Even in minute amounts the virus rapidly attacked and killed adult mice.

In the meantime in Nigeria, Dr. Donald Carey had begun the field epidemiologic investigations designed to track down the source of infection. The possibilities seemed endless—viruses, bacteria, funguses in huge numbers, places, foods, sewage, animals, and countless other potential things might be responsible for the spread. The best bet for the source of an unknown infectious disease is an animal. Under certain circumstances, many animal infections may cause disease in humans. Rabies is a common and nonlethal infection in bats that is devastating in humans and dogs. Marburg disease is normally an infection of green monkeys which first appeared in laboratory workers in Germany who were working with the monkeys. Yellow fever is also a disease of animals, as are anthrax, brucellosis, dengue, tularemia, equine encephalitis, and all the other conditions listed in table 1.2.

Carey drafted Graham Kemp to begin trapping small animals in the African bush in order to check them for the virus that had appeared in the Yale cultures. Initially, Kemp believed that yellow fever was the cause of the strange illness, but an interview with the staff in Lassa changed his mind. At Columbia Presbyterian, Penny Pinneo began to improve, clearly on the

TABLE 1.2
Some Animal Diseases Which Commonly Affect Humans

Disease	Means of Transmission to Humans
1. Anthrax	Exposure, ingestion of infected livestock
2. Bacterial food poisoning	Ingestion of contaminated meat
3. Brucellosis	Ingestion of contaminated meat, dairy products
4. Glanders	Contact with infected horses
5. Plague	Bites from infected wild animal fleas; also airborne
6. Relapsing fever	Bites from infected rodent fleas, lice
7. Shigella (dysentery)	Contact with infected primates
8. Ringworm	Contact with infected mammals, birds
9. Cryptococcosis	Contact with infected animals, especially pigeons
10. Toxoplasmosis	Contact with infected birds, mammals, especially cats
11. Swimmer's itch	Exposure to water contaminated by infected birds, rodents
12. Hydatid disease	Ingestion of eggs from infected livestock, wild animals
13. Rabies	Bite of infected mammal, especially bats and carnivores
14. Yellow fever	Bite of mosquito which has fed from infected monkey
15. Encephalitis, several types	Bite of mosquito or tick which has fed from infected bird or mammal
16. Cowpox	Contact with infected cattle
17. Lassa fever	Contact with infected rodents. Ingestion? Inhalation?
18. Cat scratch fever	Wounds, scratches inflicted by infected cat, dog

NOTE: The following publication lists 189 animal diseases which are transmitted to humans: Center for Disease Control, *Epidemiological Aspects of Some of the Zoonoses*, U.S. Department of Health, Education, and Welfare, DHEW Publication No. (CDC) 64-8182, 1973.

road to recovery. There was vast relief and the crisis seemed over. But the laboratory had discovered that the infant mice who had not reacted to the virus injections were excreting live, active viruses in their urine weeks later. These mice were highly hazardous creatures to handle, and this hazard had not been previously appreciated. In June, Jordi Casals, one of the principal investigators of the virus, became ill and began to sink rapidly. Penny Pinneo was asked if she would consider donating some of her serum, which was by now teeming with antibodies to the Lassa virus, for injection into Casals. Before the cultures confirmed that Casals indeed had Lassa fever, the serum was administered. He had been on the brink of death. Within a day, rapid improvement occurred. Despite everyone's pleasure at this, the ominous question of how he had become infected remained. Apparently, laboratory procedures were not safe enough.

The Public Health Service was also concerned. What if other travelers from Africa were to introduce this deadly disease unknowingly into the country? An effort was made to inform physicians of the situation and to keep an eye out for suspicious illnesses in incoming travelers. Knowing the danger of the virus, much of the work was transferred to the new maximum security laboratory of the Center for Disease Control in Atlanta. A few weeks later Casals was back in the laboratory, his urine now negative for virus.

By September, case reports began to filter in from various mission hospitals on the Nigerian plateau of an increasing number of admissions with fever and vague, nonspecific symptoms. Donald Carey went to the Jos plateau to investigate, along with Graham Kemp and an entomologist named Vern Lee. By the time they arrived reports of deaths and illness were pouring out of the hinterlands. Death rates were as high as 60 percent in some of the hospitals. Lee was out in the woods catching mosquitos by letting them bite his arm. This was risky, in view of the reason he was catching them. He believed they might be the source of the devastating outbreak of disease. That disease turned out to be yellow fever, not Lassa fever, and a massive yellow fever vaccination program was mounted. The Lassa virus problem was put on the back burner.

In the meantime, at Yale, a laboratory employee who had not worked with the Lassa virus became severely ill while away for the Thanksgiving weekend. A few days later he died, his body riddled with Lassa virus. No channel of infection could be identified. He had never come into contact with any of the Lassa materials. All research on the virus at Yale was instantly stopped. Other employees as well as those at the Philadelphia laboratory where his specimens had first been sent for analysis were in a panic. What if they had become infected?

In Nigeria, the yellow fever epidemic faded away. But in Jos, in December, a woman arrived at the hospital in grave condition, with nonspecific symptoms. She stayed ten days, recovered, and returned home. Within three days of return her mother and two children came down with high fever. One daughter died. None of the cases was reported to the mission hospital. A few days afterwards, cases of the same sort began to arrive at the hospital. Several died. Then, one of the hospital staff became ill and died. While performing the autopsy, Dr. Jeanette Troup who had been close to the victims of the Lassa fever outbreak earlier in the year, cut her finger with the surgical knife. By this time nineteen cases of the mysterious disease had been admitted to the Jos hospital and ten had died. Three of four staff members who had been stricken were among the dead. Careful interviews failed to identify common exposures. When news reached New York that Dr. Troup was seriously ill, Jordi Casals left immediately for the airport with two units of his now immune serum for shipment to her. It did not arrive in time.

Finally well enough to travel, Penny Pinneo returned to Nigeria with three units of immune serum for the rapidly expanding number of cases of Lassa fever. She also came with a good knowledge of Hausa, the local language, to assist the investigating team in tracking down the source of infection. Exhaustive interviewing was required to determine that all those who had become ill recently had been in the Sudan Interior Mission when the first victim had been there, but she had given a false name and address.

A program was initiated to test blood from hospitals all over sub-Saharan Africa for the presence of antibodies against Lassa virus. This would allow a determination of the distribution of the disease and, perhaps, also of its carrier animal. The infant mice in the laboratory who continued to shed live viruses throughout their lives remained vivid in the investigators' memories. These types of antibody studies are called sero-epidemiologic studies, and they permit the determination of past patterns of infection.

Eventually, the unidentified woman admitted to the Jos hospital in December was located. Blood studies confirmed that she had had Lassa fever, but they were no closer to determining the source of her infection.

Another outbreak was reported in Zorzor, Guinea. Here, as in Nigeria, all the cases seemed to be linked, but there was little indication of where the primary case had started. Sierra Leone was next. That outbreak was the biggest yet, and infections were clearly being transmitted outside the hospital. Local chiefs, though, were usually indifferent or antagonistic to the investigations. Within hours after the arrival of the investigating team in Sierra Leone, a local woman died of Lassa fever. Eight wild bush rats (*Mastomys natalensis*) had been trapped in her house. These rats were a tiny fraction of the thousands of animals that had been collected across half a dozen African nations. The dead woman's family was only one of many hundreds of similar families interviewed, tested, and examined over a period of a year and a half. It took that long just to learn the right questions and where to ask them. The end, when it finally came, was less than dramatic because of the time that had elapsed. It wasn't until several months later that these rats were finally tested and found to be filled with Lassa virus. The animal source of disease had been identified as a normally forest-dwelling rat which came into houses only when larger and more vicious house rats abandoned the premises. The cause—and the consequent measures for prevention—had at last been identified.

This is a superficial look at a true story as dramatic and mysterious as the finest mystery novel. For those interested, I recommend John Fuller's 1974 book on Lassa fever, *Fever!* Dealing with an infectious disease can be extraordinarily complex, as this book illustrates. When epidemiologists investigate the sources of noninfectious conditions such as cancer or heart disease, the multiple contributing causes of these conditions make the task all that much more difficult.

EVALUATION

Because epidemiologic methods developed as a means for inferring cause from imperfect sources of information, epidemiology's techniques have become especially applicable to the evaluation of health programs and approaches. Evaluation is simply a process in which the outcome of any planned activity is appraised against the original objectives of the activity. Although this sounds commonsensical enough, evaluation is often not considered by persons undertaking a project or program. They assume that the activity is beneficial. At the end of the program, however, a desire for more funds to continue the effort might lead to a request for information from the funding source as a demonstration that some good has been accomplished. At that point everyone scurries around trying to prove that they've been doing something useful. Retrospective evaluations of this sort are difficult, if not impossible, to accomplish reliably.

An example will clarify this issue. Suppose you are an enthusiastic supporter of community blood pressure screening. You are a health-conscious activist for the black community, a group which you know to be particularly susceptible to high blood pressure. A state agency provides you with funds to perform full-time screening activities for one year. At the end of that year you request a continuation of your support, and the agency says they need some justification that this is a good use for their money.

"Well," you tell them, "we screened 8,176 people."

"So what?" they reply.

"We found 639 people with high blood pressure," you answer proudly.

"So, big deal," they tell you. "What good did that do?"

"Well," you say, "we referred them to their doctors, and we know that high blood pressure is bad for you, and, what's more, the literature is very clear on the fact that treating people with high blood pressure reduces their risk of dying."

You are confident you've got them at that point, but they aren't biting.

"We agree that treating high blood pressure is a good thing," they say, "although that has been certain only for the last few years. However, did these people you identified get their blood pressures lowered? Did they really go to their doctors? Did their doctors give them treatment if they did go? Did they take the treatment if it was given to them?"

You are perplexed.

"How should we know?" you ask, exasperated. "We identified their high blood pressure and told them to get it treated."

The state representative says to you, shaking his head, that it is well known that simply telling people who feel well that they need to see a doctor for treatment does not lead to very high compliance rates. If your program does not lead to demonstrated reductions in blood pressure, it may very well be a total waste of money.

The state representative is correct. Many ambitious programs, conducted at great cost, have been shown to be useless when properly evaluated. Chapter 8 discusses a few of the medical practices that have bitten the dust when finally subjected to responsible evaluation. As costs of medical and health care have escalated geometrically, so have the demands for proof of efficacy, and epidemiologists have been frequently called on to design evaluation plans. I was recently hired as an evaluation consultant for a large, federally funded community health program in a major American city. A part of this program involved a liaison with the local chapter of the American Cancer Society, and a requirement of the funding agency was proper evaluation of the activities. Although there were problems in all areas, the relationship with the Cancer Society was finally terminated— largely because that group refused to allow their programs to be evaluated. As one official of that group said candidly, "We don't really want to have our programs evaluated. We know how many people we serve, how many brochures we distribute, and how many advertisements we produce. That's enough. The board would not like it if these activities were found to be ineffective."

This attitude, which is not uncommon in all walks of life, can lead to the squandering of resources in order to preserve a comfortable status quo. The official was referring to an important but little-understood difference between what are called process measures and outcome measures.

Process measures are tallies of activities performed, such as the number of people screened, the number of brochures distributed, the number of examinations performed, advertisements printed, interviews conducted, and so on. Such measures bear no relationship to the reasons that these activities are conducted, and they are useful only as a means of keeping track of whether or not work goals are being met. Outcome measures are those which directly address the reasons for conducting an activity. In the case of the blood pressure screening program, an acceptable outcome measure might be the number of people under active blood pressure treatment as a result of the screening, or, even better, the actual decline in blood pressure levels as a result of the screening program. If there were no pre-existing information confirming that a decline in blood pressure actually leads to beneficial effects on health, even this measure would be inadequate. For example, it has never been shown that treating people with borderline, asymptomatic diabetes leads to a reduction in the morbid effects of diabetes. Thus, a screening program which diagnosed diabetes, referred borderline diabetics to physicians, and made certain that diet and/or medical therapy resulted would still not have any demonstrated effectiveness. In the real world, "proof" is often hard to come by, and decisions must often be made on the basis of imperfect knowledge. Chapter 7 addresses these issues in some depth as they apply to screening programs.

VARIATION AND BIAS

A concept difficult for nonepidemiologists to understand is the difference between variation and bias. Variation means that a given measure, such as blood pressure, is not always the same when repeated under different circumstances, but that the difference is as likely to be in one direction as the next. An example of such variation is provided in a series of articles on epidemiology for the uninitiated which appeared in the *British Medical Journal* in 1978.[4]

Using death certificates which identified esophageal cancer as a cause of death, an inquiry was conducted into the validity of the diagnoses. Shown in tabular form the certificates fell into these categories.

Esophageal Cancer	Number
Diagnosed by clinician	74
Confirmed by pathologist	53
Not confirmed by pathologist	21
First diagnosed at autopsy	22

Of the seventy-four cases identified by physicians, twenty-one were in error (false positives). Of the seventy-five cases (fifty-three and twenty-two) confirmed by autopsy, twenty-two were missed by physicians (false negatives). These error rates may seem large, but so long as adequate numbers are present, mortality statistics in the population are quite accurate. The reason is that the false negatives and the false positives balance each other. So long as variation away from the "true" results is equally distributed in both directions it remains unbiased, and meaningful conclusions may be drawn from the data. This is, of course, a completely different issue from the importance of having a correct diagnosis for the care of any individual patient.

Bias is what occurs when the variation is not equally distributed, but tends to move preferentially in one direction or another. For example, if you wanted to know what percentage of the population has heart disease at any given moment (the "prevalence" of heart disease), and you stood on the street corner and asked passers-by if they had heart disease, you would have a serious problem with bias. The reason is that many people with heart disease are not able to get up and walk down the street because they are too sick. Your street sample selectively eliminates people who are sick, some of whom have heart disease, and you will very likely underestimate the prevalence of that condition.

Bias is the central issue of epidemiologic research. It occurs not only where it is expected, but also where it is not expected, and that is the major problem. There are many ways to take this unknown bias into account, and some of these are discussed in chapter 3. Fundamentally, though, all scientific investigations require confirmation, and until it is forthcoming, all results, no matter how sound they may seem, are preliminary. Epidemiology is certainly no different from other areas of investigation in this respect, but articles on health in the popular press tend to neglect the preliminary nature of such investigations because they are "newsworthy."

HEALTH AND DISEASE

A popular myth in present-day society concerns the notion that health care and disease care are the same thing, that physicians are experts in health, and that we have in the United States a superb health-care system. We speak of the need for (or arguments against) national "health" insurance to replace private "health" insurance. But the maintenance of health and the treatment of disease are separate endeavors that might be likened to routine maintenance of an automobile in comparison to repair of damaged parts. Routine maintenance is not nearly as complex or as difficult as repair, and it is enormously important to preventing the need for repair. It is as simple—and as complex—as sound nutrition, regular exercise, minimal stress, not smoking, and a few other such basic behaviors. If you know how to do an excellent valve job when the need arises, but fail to understand the need for routine oil changes and periodic tune-ups, you would have a car that gave you a great deal of trouble.

Our health care system is precisely in that situation. We are as good at trouble shooting as it is possible to be, given the limits of modern technology, but our maintenance procedures are a disaster. We are so far off the mark that we even call the care of disease "health care." We have enormous organizations which provide high levels of medical care at relatively low cost, called health maintenance organizations (HMOs), but they almost totally lack health maintenance activities. National health insurance bills in Congress, regardless of author, contain no provisions for health, only for the treatment of disease. What happens to the diseased individual who has been made well if the ultimate cause of the disease has not been addressed?

In 1818 the French physician Louis Rene Villerme gave up his medical practice in despair because of the ineffectiveness of medical practice. In 1948 John Ryle resigned his post as regius professor of medicine at Cambridge saying:

Thirty years of my life have been spent as a student and teacher of clinical medicine. In these thirty years I have watched disease in the ward being studied more and more thoroughly—if not always more thoughtfully—through the high power of the microscope; disease in man being investigated by more and more elaborate techniques and, on the whole, more and more mechanically. . . . The morbid "material" of the hospital ward consists very largely—if we exclude the emergencies—of end-result conditions for which, as a rule, only a limited amount of relief repays the long stay, the patient investigation, and the anxious expectancy of the sick man or woman. With aetiology—the first essential for prevention—and with prevention itself the majority of physicians and surgeons have curiously little concern.[5]

These physicians, like those who developed the epidemiologic method whose work is discussed in the next chapter, were frustrated by the fact that their chosen profession had somehow let them down. For them, the drama of medicine was unable to eclipse the fact that it was frequently unable to deal with problems on a larger scale and in the long run. Its solutions were too often transient or inadequate. The remedy is not so much better technology as a change in philosophy.

The physician receives little training in nutrition, in human sexuality, in counseling and interpersonal relationships, in behavior change, or in addressing and identifying the causes of the conditions that he or she treats. Other than routine immunizations, there is little in the doctor's black bag that addresses prevention rather than cure. The physician is, in other words, trained to treat disease.

That physicians lack training in health care would not necessarily be inappropriate if the public and physicians themselves recognized this limitation and referred their clients to other, more relevant professionals to deal with those issues. Unfortunately, the public continues to ask questions of doctors which they have absolutely no training or facility for answering, and doctors, unaware that their training has been so inadequate in these areas, continue to answer them. The result is that the world's most expensive medical care system exists in a nation where health status is, for an industrialized nation, mediocre at best. Table 1.3 presents a comparison of mean life expectancies at birth in 1976 for thirteen industrialized nations which keep comparable records. The United States ranks seventh in life

TABLE 1.3
Life Expectancy at Birth According to Sex:
Selected Countries, 1976[1]
(Data are based on reporting by countries)

Country	MALE Remaining life expectancy in years	Rank	FEMALE Remaining life expectancy in years	Rank
Canada	69.6	8	77.1	6
United States	69.0	11	76.7	7
Sweden	72.2	2	78.1	2
England and Wales	69.7	7	75.8	10
Netherlands	71.6	4	78.1	2
German Democratic Republic	68.9	12	74.5	13
German Federal Republic	68.1	13	74.7	11
France	69.5	9	77.6	4
Switzerland	71.7	3	78.3	1
Italy	69.9	6	76.1	9
Israel[2]	71.0	5	74.7	11
Japan	72.3	1	77.6	4
Australia	69.3	10	76.4	8

[1]Data for Canada, France, and Italy refer to 1974; data for the German Federal Republic, Israel, and Australia refer to 1975.

[2]Jewish population only.

SOURCES: World Health Organization, *World Health Statistics, 1978,* Vol. 1, Geneva, World Health Organization, 1978; United Nations, *Demographic Yearbook 1976,* Publication no. ST/ESA/STAT/SER.R/4, New York, United Nations, 1977; "Final Mortality Statistics, 1976," *Monthly Vital Statistics Report,* Vol. 26, No. 12, supplement 2, U.S. Department of Health, Education, and Welfare, Publication no. (PHS) 78-1120, March 30, 1978.

expectancy for women and eleventh for men, despite the fact that its health care expenditures per person far exceed those of any other nation. I would hasten to add that life expectancy is a rather poor indicator of the quality of life in any given society, but there are few international yardsticks other than life expectancy which permit cross-cultural comparisons. One might select crime indices (the United States has the world's highest rates of violent crimes during peacetime) or the incidence of depression (which currently appears to have reached epidemic proportions in the United States) as other measures of quality of life. This is not meant to be an indictment of the medical care system. It offers superb medical treatment, probably the best in the world. It does not, however, deal with the causes of disease, with prevention, with the well person in hopes of keeping him well, or with what makes people have fulfilling and satisfying lives.

Many disciplines do deal with these issues, and the epidemiologist is involved in some of them. Table 1.1 is taken from the previously mentioned article on definitions of epidemiology. Running through all of these definitions is the notion that epidemiology deals somehow with the distribution of diseases in populations. This reflects an historical background more than a discipline. That is to say, epidemiology is a method for studying the patterns of occurrence of disease in populations, a disease-detective approach which results in the ability to infer cause from these patterns. In fact, the methods of epidemiology have been used by social psychologists, by medical anthropologists, and even by economists to study the causes of observed events. It is surprising to collaborate with these people and find that, beneath their own particular jargon, they are using the same techniques I use to infer cause and develop methods of "prevention."

Because epidemiology has so much in common with these other disciplines, it might be more useful to think of it as a specialized method of investigation rather than as a distinct body of homogenous information such as chemistry or biology. This method has as a foundation the techniques for comparing numbers in a meaningful fashion. Scientists of all sorts encounter this need, but in most sciences true experimentation can be performed. The chemist can control precisely the reagents going into his test tubes. The biologist can control the conditions under which he studies life in the laboratory, and the physiologist can study his plants and animals under uniform circumstances, even down to breeding genetically identical strains. But when people are studied, ethical considerations demand alternative approaches. The stringent requirements of laboratory experimentation cannot be applied to humans, as will be discussed in detail later. Instead, rules of inference have been worked out which involve strict control over how information is collected and analyzed. (Unfortunately, neither the lay public nor the majority of physicians are trained in these skills, and the consequences of this lack are discussed in chapter 6.) Epidemiologic conclusions are based on comparisons of rates of occurrence of various events in different populations or groups of people.

Epidemiology provides a means for identifying modifiable causes of disease on the specific to the general level. The "cause" assumes a broader, more general implication, as is discussed in the chapter on transmission of diseases. Cause becomes anything that can serve to interrupt the spread of disease. Thus, in the epidemiologic sense, food poisoning is caused not only by staphylococci (bacteria), but also by inadequate refrigeration. Tuberculosis is caused by poor sanitation as well as by a microorganism.

THE USES OF EPIDEMIOLOGY

In his classic work, *The Uses of Epidemiology*, J. N. Morris discussed the practical applications of the science. These applications are broad and overlap substantially with other disciplines. Epidemiology is, perhaps, the most interdisciplinary of the medical sciences, since in one way or another it involves work in nearly every branch of the biological sciences.

Epidemiology is used to study the historical background of health and disease in order to arrive at projections of future health issues. It is the principal means for assessing the level of general community health, identifying groups of persons at especially high risk for certain diseases, and measuring the impact of programs designed to reduce that risk. Most fundamentally, it is used to search for the causes of both illness and wellness, and to plot strategies for improving well-being.

In a similar vein, epidemiology can be used to identify the specific probability that a given individual will suffer from a disease. Such information permits individuals at high risk to take early preventive action and so avoid becoming ill. It is also used to describe the entire biology of illnesses and, thus, to see the course of disease as a whole, rather than as a limited phenomenon. This wholistic view of disease facilitates the identification of physical or chemical processes which can be used to interrupt transmission and also diagnose and treat cases at early stages in the course of illness. Finally, epidemiology is being used increasingly to evaluate the operations of health services with the aim of providing the maximum of care at a minimum cost.[6] Certainly, these uses overlap each other to some degree. But they succeed better than any definition in describing what epidemiology is all about.

Because of the difficulties in making decisions on the basis of the kinds of information that can be gathered from large groups of human beings, epidemiologists have developed some fundamental ideas about judging the usefulness of information. These ideas turn out to be highly useful tools for judging the credence of almost any statement which is based on the use of data (statistics) to draw conclusions. Statistics do not lie (assuming the data are accurately collected), but they can mislead if their meaning is misunderstood. The remainder of this book provides the reader with a few basic tools for making judgments in the face of masses of information. Underlying the use of all of these tools, however, is the idea that it is important to maintain a careful balance between openness to new ideas and healthy skepticism.

Chapter 2
A Brief History of the Field

Epidemiologists Who Never Knew That That's What They Were

When the Greeks have flooded us with their literature, and especially their physicians, they will ruin everything for us.

—Cato

Perhaps the first epidemiologist who dared to publish his findings was Hippocrates,[1] who pointed out that it was considerably less healthy to live in low places than it was to live in high ones, laying the blame on bad air and water. Nevertheless, people continued to live in low places, possibly because Hippocrates neglected to adjust his findings for age, sex, and socioeconomic status. Since there were no other epidemiologists around to criticize his methods, he was spared castigations in the letters-to-the-editor column, which would inevitably accompany such a faux pas in our modern age.

One can hardly say that epidemiology "caught on" after this initial foray into the world of scientific publishing, for it was nearly two

thousand years before iron-fisted editors could be induced to
permit another publication in the fledgling field. John Graunt
was a rather antisocial Englishman who lived in London during
the seventeenth century, and it was his meticulous examination
of apparently useless information that led in large part to the
modern sciences of epidemiology and vital statistics.

JOHN GRAUNT

In his major work, *Natural and Political Observations Made
upon the Bills of Mortality*, Graunt laid the foundation for the
use of vital statistics as a means of understanding changes in the
health of a population and for planning ways of coping with the
problems of urban areas in a less than haphazard fashion.[2]

Graunt was both intrigued and puzzled to learn that, from
1592 to 1594 and then regularly from December 1603, the English crown published weekly Bills of Mortality which included
a record of burials, christenings, and causes of death for each
parish in London and the surrounding area. Although this practice had continued nearly seventy years when he became interested in it, he could find no use to which the information was
put or reason for its collection. Annual summaries were duti-
fully issued each year on the Thursday before Christmas Day,
filed in the archives, and promptly forgotten. Obviously, government's penchant for collecting data that may be useful at
some time, even if it isn't now, is not a new one.

Graunt saw some potential uses. He spent several reclusive
years tabulating and estimating, identifying healthy years and
sick years, and trying to find characteristics that were unique to
each. Table 2.1 lists the causes of death for the year 1632.
Clearly, disease classification systems have changed somewhat
since that time, but the data are still highly revealing. The leading cause of death is a complex of infant diseases referred to as
"chrisomes, and infants" (infant deaths, especially due to diar-
rhea). Next comes consumption (wasting diseases, primarily
tuberculosis and cancer), then fevers.

TABLE 2.1
The Diseases, and Casualties this year being 1632

445—Abortive, and Stillborn	4—Gout
1—Affrighted	11—Grief
628—Aged	43—Jaundies
43—Ague	8—Jawfaln
17—Apoplex, and Meagrom	74—Impostume
1—Bit with a mad dog	46—Kil'd by several accidents
3—Bleeding	38—King's Evil
348—Bloody flux, scowring, and flux	2—Lethargie
	87—Livergrown
26—Brused, Issues, sores, and ulcers	5—Lunatique
	15—Made away themselves
5—Burnt, and Scalded	80—Measles
9—Burst, and Rupture	7—Murthered
10—Cancer, and wolf	7—Over-laid, and starved at nurse
1—Canker	
171—Childbed	25—Palsie
2268—Chrisomes, and Infants	1—Piles
55—Cold, and Cough	8—Plague
56—Colick, Stone, and Strangury	13—Planet
	36—Pleurisie, and Spleen
1797—Consumption	38—Purples, and Spotted Fever
241—Convulsion	
5—Cut of the Stone	7—Quinsie
6—Dead in the Street, and starved	98—Rising of the Lights
	1—Sciatica
267—Dropsie, and Swelling	9—Scurvey, and Itch
34—Drowned	62—Suddenly
18—Executed, and prest to death	86—Surfet
	6—Swine Pox
7—Falling Sickness	470—Teeth
1108—Fever	40—Thrush, and sore mouth
13—Fistula	13—Tympany
531—Flocks, and Small Pox	34—Tissick
12—French Pox	1—Vomiting
5—Gangrene	27—Worms

	4994—Males		4932—Males	8—Whereof,
Christened	4590—Females	Buried	4603—Females	of the
	9584—In all		9535—In all	Plague

993—Increased in the Burials in the 122 Parishes, and at the Pest-house this year

266—Decreased of the Plague in the 122 Parishes, and at the Pest-house this year

He was also able to identify major plague years—1592–1593, 1603, 1625, and 1636. He developed the concepts of rates and proportions as better measures of health status than absolute numbers, and used proportionate mortality (the fraction of all deaths due to a given cause) for plague as a means of identifying the worst plague epidemics. He correctly pointed out the uses of such data for civic planning, for assessing major health problems, for correcting tax and military draft records, and for identifying population and health disproportions between districts.

Graunt was, like many investigators, quite defensive about the value of his work. In his conclusion to the treatise he states:

> It may now be asked, to what purpose tends all this laborious buzzling, and groping? . . . To this I might answer in general by saying, that those, who cannot apprehend the reason of these Enquiries, are unfit to trouble themselves to ask them.

He also provides a long list of reasons for collecting and analyzing the data, and one of them is especially worth noting:

> . . . there is much pleasure in deducing so many abstruse, and unexpected inferences out of these poor despised Bills of Mortality; and in building upon that ground, which hath lain waste these eighty years. And there is pleasure in doing something new, though never so little, without pestering the World with voluminous Transcriptions.

From these humble beginnings one might trace the roots of vital statistics, survey research, and epidemiology. The intellectual revolution of the seventeenth and eighteenth centuries was such that this seed did not long lie ungerminated. A history so brief as this must, of necessity, leave out many contributors, especially those who wrote in other languages and have not been translated into English. But several observations by seventeenth century English physicians were unprecedented in their health effects on society and in the sophistication of the methodology used.

JAMES LIND

It is fair to say that few modern clinicians save even a small fraction of the lives and ease as much suffering as James Lind and George Baker, whose accomplishments were notable particularly because they dealt with prevention rather than cure of diseases.

Lind became interested in scurvy, a disease which devastated navies and crews of commercial vessels. Scurvy is a particularly painful affliction which produces swollen, putrid gums, poor healing of wounds, contractions and spasms of muscles, swelling of the legs, and a variety of other problems. It regularly occurred in the course of long sea voyages, but not on short ones. It almost always cleared up rapidly (among the survivors, that is) upon reaching port.

The cause of scurvy was not understood at the time. It was often attributed to the ill effects of large amounts of sea salt. Lind noted many inconsistencies with this theory. First, he collected large numbers of instances where scurvy affected persons far from the sea. Armies were especially vulnerable in the winter. There were outbreaks among German troops in Hungary, for example, about the time Lind was doing his research. He further discovered that besieged garrisons had outbreaks, as did isolated settlements in northern climates during winter. He specified latitudes north of 60 degrees as being greatly at risk and documented these claims with examples of winter outbreaks in Iceland, Greenland, Russia, and elsewhere. His research was painstaking and thorough, not a characteristic approach of the times. He developed the concept of "predisposing causes" of disease, conditions which enhance susceptibility without being direct causes of disease, and he recognized that illness results from a variety of factors and is seldom the result of any single influence. He examined seamen's diets in minute detail and became convinced at an early stage that an inadequate diet was the principal cause of scurvy.

> It is demonstrable from the appearance of the calamity in every part of the world, that no state of air whatever is capable of producing it, without the concurrence of gross viscid diet, and abstinence from green vegetables. I have known the Channel fleet bury a hundred men in a cruise, and land a thousand more quite rotten in the scurvy; yet among the number, there was not an officer, not even a petty officer.[3]

Lind's recommendations were straightforward: Eat greens. He even suggested that, in difficult situations, sailors should pull the seaweed off the hull of the ship and eat them. Although he had never heard of vitamin C (a deficiency of which produces scurvy) and he lacked any understanding of the physiological basis for the need for greens, Lind was able to suggest an effective preventive measure. This was adopted some years later by the British navy, which issued rations of limes to its sailors as a means for preventing the scurvy. This earned English seamen the nickname "Limeys," which they retain to this day. His preventive advice saved thousands of lives and tens of thousands of miserable cases of scurvy. By examining the factors associated with the outbreak of disease in an effort to determine an effective means for preventing the disease, he also ushered in the era of modern epidemiology, a science which strives to prevent disease by studying those factors associated with the occurrence of health and illness.

GEORGE BAKER

George Baker's name is even less familiar to modern readers than is Lind's. This may be attributed to Baker's total success in his most important endeavor: elimination of the endemial colic of Devonshire. In 1768, Baker published *An Essay Con-*

cerning the Cause of the Endemial Colic of Devonshire, a
work which began with a complaint often voiced in present
times:

> A very small acquaintance with the writings of physicians is suf-
> ficient to convince us, that much labour and ingenuity has been
> most unprofitably bestowed on the investigation of remote and
> obscure causes; while those, which are obvious and evident . . .
> which must necessarily be acknowledged as soon as stumbled
> upon, have been too frequently overlooked and disregarded.[4]

Baker described the endemial colic as "a malady, so formida-
ble as well in its immediate effects, as in its more distant consequences, it is an office of humanity, as much as possible, to
prevent." The colic was a frequently fatal and severely painful
intestinal affliction, largely limited to adult male inhabitants of
Devonshire. It had a seasonal distribution, peaking in the au-
tumn of each year, and had been associated by others with the
production of the hard cider which made Devonshire famous.
But Baker was not satisfied with hearsay. He recognized immediately that many people in other parts of England drank copi-
ous amounts of cider without developing the colic. Further, he
noted similarities between the symptoms of Devonshire colic
and lead poisoning.

To confirm his ideas, he conducted a series of five experiments that had grown out of the results of his population-based
studies. He confirmed the presence of lead in Devonshire cider
and the absence of lead in cider from other locations, and noted
that the use of lead in fermentation vats had become common
practice about the time that the colic first became a problem.
His solution, phrased in polite, eighteenth century English
reads:

> May not I presume to hope, that the present discovery of a poi-
> son, which has for many years exerted its virulant effects on the
> inhabitants of Devonshire, incorporated with their daily liquor,

unobserved, and unsuspected, may be esteemed by those, who have power, and who have opportunities to remove the source of so much mischief, to be an object worthy of their most serious attention?

Baker's solution—get the lead out—resulted in the virtual elimination of the deadly colic within a short time. Those who truly solve problems are usually forgotten since nothing remains to remind us of the work they have done. Presumably, the modern elimination of smallpox, which depended on the development of a technique for identification and containment of outbreaks (the vaccine had been around for more than one hundred fifty years), will lead to similar obscurity for D. A. Henderson and his colleagues. We have already forgotten that less than twenty years ago more than a million people died of that disease every year.

PERCIVAL POTT

One of the first English writers to discuss occupation-related disease was an English surgeon named Percival Pott. In 1740 he published an essay, "Cancer Scroti," in which he noted that chimney sweeps had an inordinately high rate of cancer of the scrotum.[5] This was probably the first medical notation of the carcinogenic potential of burned organic material. (Cigarette smoking, of course, provides a more timely example of this phenomenon, since there are no longer enough chimney sweeps around to study.) If Potts' methods were crude, his conclusions were not, and his work, too, provided a clear and obvious solution to a problem for which there was no effective therapy.

PETER PANUM

It remained for a young Danish physician, Peter L. Panum, to present the first thoroughly sound analysis of a disease outbreak.[6] In 1846, Panum was dispatched by his government to investigate a devastating outbreak of measles in the Faroe Islands, a group of seventeen cold, windy islands in the North Atlantic. Panum's bleak description describes the territory:

> The vegetation of the country is limited to grass, small herbs, barley and potatoes. Trees or bushes do not thrive, frankly speaking, and even the efforts which certain government officials have made to promote, by the use of high enclosures, the fostering of currant and gooseberry bushes, willow and serviceberry bushes, have not given any very cheering results. It seems to be less the temperature than the mists, blended with saline and other particles of sea water, in conjunction with the powerful winds, that hinders their growth.

Because the Faroes were so isolated, disease which existed at low or endemic levels in the European population tended to be absent from the Faroes for many years, only to break out with ferocious intensity when imported from the mainland. At the time, nothing was known about the cause of measles. The germ theory of disease was barely a glimmer in the minds of a few "crackpot" scientists, and population-based concepts of epidemiology were crude and inexact. Panum was undeterred by these problems. The inexperienced Dane carefully tracked down every traceable case of measles, interviewed family and neighbors, and put his answers together with careful age stratification that told him a great deal about the disease.

He used rates instead of numbers for his figures, a practice which allowed him to make what may be the first cross-cultural mortality comparisons (between the Faroes and Denmark) and permitted him to observe the age differentials in death rates. He accurately calculated the incubation period of the disease, noted the existence of immunity in the older individuals who had been resident during the last outbreak, and estimated the relation between age and risk of death from measles. Although he did not determine any specific methods for preventing measles, he did make effective recommendations with respect to quarantine measures that would prevent the spread of the disease once it broke out. These were important, because measles can be a deadly disease in nonresistant populations. More important, he demonstrated that measles is a contagious disease that does not arise spontaneously. He even suggested that it was caused by a living organism. He concluded accurately that measles was not spread "miasmatically," but rather was communicated from person to person through contact or through contact with objects recently touched by an infected individual. These concepts of the etiology and spread of a disease were derived, like Baker's cure for colic, without benefit of laboratory science. Panum relied solely on observations of the behavior of disease in populations.

JOHN SNOW

If any man can be called the father of modern epidemiology, it is the English physician John Snow. He was best known in his own time as the physician who administered chloroform to Queen Victoria at the birth of her son Prince Leopold, an occasion which brought the wonders of anesthesia to widespread public attention. But Snow's principal work centered around the devastating epidemics of cholera which swept through London every few years.

Perhaps the worst of these epidemics was centered in the St. James' district of Westminster in 1854. Snow had already done considerable research on previous epidemics and felt that his understanding of the nature of the malady was taking shape. Within a ten-day period, more than five hundred persons, most of whom lived near the area, died of the disease. For epidemiologists, this is probably the single best-known outbreak of disease in history, the notoriety occasioned by Snow's masterful analysis of the cause of the epidemic and the action he took to stop it.

Snow's previous work had led him to believe that contaminated water was somehow involved in most epidemics of cholera. He developed the notion of plotting the residences of cases on a map of London in order to determine their geographic relationship to one another. (This technique is still widely practiced among epidemiologists.) The few cases who did not live near the outbreak were especially important, since interviews inevitably determined that they had visited the affected area just before becoming ill.

Shortly after beginning his investigation, Snow began to suspect that a popular pump on Broad Street, highly reputed for the excellent quality of its water, might be implicated. It seemed "that there was no other circumstance or agent common to the circumscribed locality in which the sudden increase in cholera occurred."[7]

On the evening of September 7, he appeared before the Board of Guardians to explain his case. Although many members expressed disbelief that so fine and clear a water as that from the Broad Street pump could contain the seeds of such calamity, or indeed, that contaminated water, even if clearly dirty, should cause the cholera, they nevertheless agreed to remove the pump handle on the following morning. Within a few days the epidemic had abated.

Now, Snow was nobody's fool. He had studied enough epidemics to know that characteristically there is a rapid rise in cases, a brief plateau, then a rapid decline, which occurs because there are no more susceptible persons in the neighborhood to catch the disease. When the pump handle was removed, the peak of the epidemic curve had already been reached. The subsequent decline in number of cases was inevitable, pump or no pump. Snow knew this and used this private knowledge judiciously to support his case.

As meticulous and potentially life-saving as Snow's work had been, it was not until long after his death in 1858 that the hygienic measures he recommended were finally adopted and the periodic cholera epidemics ended. Henry Whitehead, a minister and contemporary of Snow, began by opposing Snow's views and ended as one of his great supporters. He recalled a prophetic comment that Snow had made to him: "You and I may not live to see the day, and my name may be forgotten when it comes, but the time will arrive when great outbreaks of cholera will be things of the past; and it is the knowledge of the way in which the disease is propagated which will cause them to disappear."[8] This early recognition that one need not understand the specific pathophysiology of a disease in order to halt its spread laid the groundwork for the coming public health revolution of the early twentieth century, which produced dramatic improvements in life expectancy primarily from hygienic measures.

Except among epidemiologists, John Snow is almost unknown. A small plaque marks the spot on Broad Street where the pump once stood, and next to it is the John Snow Pub, an ordinary English tavern which commemorates, in name at least, one of the outstanding medical detectives of all time. Recently an American epidemiologist friend of mine visited the pub and asked the bartender about the origin of the establishment's name. The puzzled barman shook his head and allowed as how he wasn't really certain, but thought maybe the bloke was an old-time politician or something.

JOSEPH GOLDBERGER

If Snow defined the use of the epidemiologic method in understanding infectious diseases, an American, Joseph Goldberger, was the first to successfully apply scientific epidemiology to a noninfectious disease. He did this somewhat backhandedly, since he began his work thinking that pellagra was highly infectious.

Pellagra occurs throughout the world, and by the beginning of this century it had become an especially serious problem in the rural South. Mental institutions were most likely to have outbreaks of the illness, and the lack of attention many mentally ill people often pay to hygiene was thought to facilitate the spread of the condition. It is characterized by a painfully sore and reddened tongue, gastrointestinal disturbances, skin eruptions, and defects in nerve functions. It may be fatal.

Like Lind so many years earlier, Goldberger was struck by the fact that the distribution of pellagra cases was strange for an infectious illness. Institutionalized patients frequently became diseased, but staff almost never did. Through standard, tedious epidemiologic investigation, he managed to determine that the single characteristic shared by institutions and free-living regions where the disease was common was a similar diet, one very high in corn and corn products. Goldberger became so convinced that this terrible malady was in fact a manifestation of nutritional deficiency that he set up a series of experiments using himself as well as prisoners and orphaned children as subjects. He fed fecal material from infected persons to healthy individuals and determined that pellagra did not result. He produced pellagra in some persons by providing diets similar to those served by most mental institutions and then showed that meat, milk, and vegetables could lead to recovery from the disease.

We now know that a deficiency in the B vitamin, niacin, is responsible for pellagra, but that the situation is not simple. Where coexisting disease or deficiencies of other B vitamins occur, the likelihood of developing pellagra is greatly increased. Of all grains, corn is about the poorest in niacin content, a fact which explains why high corn consumption was associated with the disease.

THE DIFFICULTIES
OF PIONEERING

Goldberger's success in convincing the world of the cause of pellagra saved uncounted lives and suffering, and because that success was so complete, his accomplishment, like Baker's, has been largely forgotten. But it brought to an increasingly scientific and technologic world the tools and techniques for studying large groups of people to answer questions which cannot be directly addressed by studying individuals. Those responsible for the vast increase in life expectancy in the eighteenth and nineteenth centuries were not primarily medical practitioners. They were public health investigators like Snow, Baker, and Goldberger, who showed how to prevent the spread of epidemic disease. They were observers and comparers of alternative practices in groups, such as the Viennese obstetrician Semmelweis, who discovered to his horror that obstetrical practices were producing high maternal mortality rates, and Lister, who found that sepsis and death in his hospital were vastly reduced through aseptic practices. And they are sanitarians who, without notice or fanfare, see to it that the water we drink and the food we eat are safe for consumption. These are the authors of our good health.

It is worth reflecting on the difficulties most of these pioneers encountered in having their ideas accepted, even in the face of overwhelming evidence. It has been noted that Snow was long dead before his ideas and approaches were used to prevent cholera. Semmelweis was hounded out of Vienna, went to Budapest, and finally committed suicide in his anguish over the fact that his colleagues were killing their patients by utterly rejecting his easily demonstrable theories. Goldberger was reduced to eating large amounts of human excrement as a final proof to his doubters that pellagra was not infectious.

New ideas are almost never accepted through a gradual process of trial and error. Rather, the old generation gradually dies off, leaving a new generation open to the new idea. Scientists' resistance to scientific discovery is an old problem which is still very much with us.[9] Galileo was forced to recant his theory that the earth moves around the sun. Max Planck, the great physicist, could not get his professors at the University of Munich to even consider his revolutionary ideas. Gregor Mendel's achievement of determining how genes are inherited was totally ignored for more than forty years after he published his studies.

Scientists, like everyone else, have an innate resistance to new ideas. Scientific exactness easily slips into rationalized human rigidity. It is not enough for the Snows and Linds to tell us how to prevent an illness. We must be able to hear what they are saying, and we must be able to separate it from the baseless advice of charlatans and misguided medical advisers. The remainder of this book should help the reader do just that.

Chapter 3
Populations and Peoples

What the Few Can Learn from the Many

The level of public health corresponds to the degree to which the means and responsibility for coping with illnesses are distributed among the total population.

—Ivan Illich

When they first appeared on the market, birth control pills were enthusiastically embraced by millions of women who were uncomfortable with the messiness and not infrequent failures of conventional methods of preventing pregnancy. Appropriate laboratory studies had failed to demonstrate any harmful side effects. But, women were usually told that they should not use the new pills for more than five years, since so little was known of long-term effects. The greatest concern about potential long-term effects centered around cancer of the breast, cervix, and uterus, because these organs are strongly influenced by hormones. Breast cancer, for one, may accelerate or regress depending on the estrogen content of the blood stream.

It is 1963. You are an internist in private practice in New Orleans, Louisiana. It is Saturday night and you have been enjoying some Dixieland behind the cracked and dirty windows of Preservation Hall. Afterward, you stroll over to the French Market intending to pick up some French doughnuts at the Morning Call, a barren, undecorated piece of old New Orleans which reeks of atmosphere. First, though, you call your answering service to check in. There is an urgent call for you. One of your patients, Mrs. Thibidoux, a thirty-six-year-old housewife from Metairie, has been admitted to Ochsner Foundation Hospital with severe precordial chest pain. The admitting physician thinks she has suffered a heart attack. Sighing, you return to your car and drive through the Garden District to River Road, turn north, and follow the Mississippi levee to the hospital. You doubt the diagnosis. Young women seldom have heart attacks unless they have congenital or long-standing heart problems.

When you arrive, you change your mind. The electrocardiogram shows classic signs of anterior wall infarction. You keep the woman sedated and at rest for several weeks—standard treatment for the time. Eventually, she returns home feeling well. You are puzzled by the case but not concerned; after all, your patient recovered her health. Six months later Mrs. Thibidoux is found dead in her bathtub. Your assumption is that she died of a second heart attack which probably resulted from some undetected congenital defect. You know you did the best that could be done, and, being used to death, put it out of your mind. In the context of the time, it seems irrelevant that Mrs. Thibidoux smoked two packs of cigarettes a day and had been taking birth control pills for eighteen months, and you certainly were unaware that the dose of estrogen in her birth control pills was nearly ten times greater than it needed to be to reliably prevent pregnancy.

This vignette illustrates the vast chasm that separates medical treatment from investigation of cause and prevention of illness. As the treating physician you did everything properly, and, given the medical knowledge of the time, there is nothing you might have done to prevent the death of Mrs. Thibidoux. Because others were looking not at individuals but at patterns of occurrence, the death of one Cajun woman helped to prevent other such deaths which might have occurred years later.

Birth control pills were a significant innovation. Never had such a large number of healthy persons taken a medication on such a regular basis for so long a time. The experience of women taking birth control pills was subjected to enormous epidemiologic scrutiny. After ten years of widespread use it became gradually clear that women who took birth control pills were more likely to have heart attacks, stroke, and depression than women who did not. Still, these events were rare, even among women taking the pills. It further became known that the pills could effectively prevent pregnancy in much lower doses. Later it was recognized that women who smoked cigarettes were at greater risk for heart disease and stroke when they took birth control pills. As a consequence of these findings, the hormone doses in the pills were reduced markedly, and these newer, safer pills were taken by fewer women. Doctors began to advise women who smoked not to take birth control pills.

No clinical physician treating individual patients could ever have discovered the importance of these changes. The chances are small that any single doctor ever saw more than one case like Mrs. Thibidoux's, and most saw none. The use of large numbers of cases reduced to statistical distributions is the only means for determining the unknown cause of many events. Frequently, though, people try to draw conclusions about cause in other ways.

TESTIMONIAL EVIDENCE

Why couldn't Mrs. Thibidoux's doctor have simply put two and two together? After all, she had a rare disease and was taking these new pills. Surely, there was a relationship. If you had talked to Mrs. Thibidoux before her death, she would have told you why she had the heart attack. She had been born in the bayous, a strange world for most Americans. Her sister, who disliked her intensely for reasons we won't go into, practiced voodoo. Mrs. Thibidoux knew that her heart attack was her sister's doing. Mr. Thibidoux, on the other hand, was certain that his wife's recent discovery of frozen foods was responsible. For some reason, only a few months before her first attack, she had stopped using fresh ingredients and had piled her freezer full of frozen foods which tasted inferior and were obviously bad for the heart. Mr. Thibidoux knew a number of other women who had gotten sick after using frozen foods. This issue will be discussed in more detail elsewhere in this book. Suffice to say that testimonials are not reliable. The world is large, and one can find a large number of people to whom the most bizarre events have occurred. They all have personal explanations. The vast majority are wrong. It once seemed logical that the earth was flat, that pus helped wounds heal, that bloodletting cured most ills, and that pellagra was caused by a germ. In Ethiopia it is still widely believed that gonorrhea is caused by urinating in the moonlight. There are lots of anecdotes to support each of these notions.

EVIDENCE OF TRENDS

It might have been possible to identify the risk of birth control pills by examining trends in heart disease among young women. If the rate of heart disease rose when the pills came into use, doesn't that suggest a relationship? This approach is tempting to many. It has more "scientific" appeal than do testimonials. It uses grouped data to draw a conclusion. But, it is faulty. Stomach cancer has declined dramatically in this country since the early 1940s. No cause for this decline has been identified. It would be a simple matter to select the year the decline began and note every unique thing about that year. I am sure there were hundreds, perhaps thousands, as there are every year. Then, depending on your biases, you might ascribe the decline in stomach cancer to any of those things. Many people have used exactly that approach in ascribing the decline in deaths due to cervical cancer to the widespread use of Pap smears. The fact that the decline began twenty years before Pap smears were invented doesn't deter them in the least. Further, what if there is a delay in effect? It is generally recognized that cigarettes require fifteen to twenty years to produce a lung cancer. If you don't know what the lag period is, or even if it exists, you might ascribe a change in trends to any event at any time prior to that change.

Trends are useful in that they tell us where our problems lie and how they are likely to change in the future. They do not tell us anything about cause and effect.

THE CONTROLLED STUDY

Appropriately performed epidemiologic studies include some form of control group. The different types of studies and their respective reliabilities at demonstrating cause are discussed in chapter 5. Two principal factors interfere with reasonable interpretations of such studies. First, few people have been trained to recognize the differences between good and bad studies or to understand that no single epidemiologic or statistical investigation ever, by itself, *proves* that a given disease is caused by a given factor. Consistency of findings among properly performed studies that are, in fact, comparable, leads to confidence in understanding. Second, studies which have outcomes that are considered undesirable by vested interests are often the subject of confusing campaigns both criticizing their results and presenting data from inadequate studies that contradict them. Recently, Congress issued guidelines for epidemiologic studies that deal with environmental issues, because legislators were confused by contradictions in the various studies they were asked to review. The guidelines themselves are inadequate and needlessly rigid. They will impair, rather than assist, good research, and they will not end the contradictions because they don't deal with the underlying issues.

A study at Johns Hopkins University of the occupational hazards of working in an industry will inevitably have different results than one conducted by the industry itself. Unless legislators either learn to distinguish good from bad research or at least appoint and listen to advisers who can do so, they will continue to be confused by conflicting results and testimony.

Controlled studies of millions of women taking birth control pills compared to millions of similar women not taking the pills led to the recognition that certain diseases occurred with greater frequency among the pill-using women. In both groups the risk of most of these conditions was small. The vast majority of pill users also remained healthy. Public health is dependent on the ability of epidemiologic investigators to be able to make such comparisons.

SOCIAL OBLIGATIONS AND THE RIGHT TO PRIVACY

Modern societies are exposed to thousands of drugs, chemicals, sounds, and radiations which are unique to our times. We have no past experience with most of these substances and do not understand their long-range effects on the human organism or how they may interact with each other. Most of them are probably harmless. A few are already known to be deadly. A new drug may appear promising, but have serious consequences when taken by persons who are also taking another drug which interacts with it. A new chemical with widespread practical uses may cause some rare disease in workers exposed to it, in the manner that polyvinyl chloride causes liver cancer.

Our age is sufficiently technological that it is unreasonable to expect that these exposures will cease. Instead, we must be vigilant in our observations of their effects. In the past, medical researchers have occasionally abused the rights of the subjects of their studies. Politicians have abused their constituents, corporate officers their stockholders, and clergymen their congregations. In the past fifteen years a healthy movement in medical ethics has emerged to assure that medical research does not interfere with the rights of citizens. This movement to protect the subjects of human research is a desirable and useful phenomenon. Unfortunately, it has also spawned abuses of its own. In the name of protecting the right to privacy, some hospitals have refused qualified researchers access to medical records without a separate signed consent form for each use of the record. This sounds reasonable, but it is impractical for epidemiologic research. The studies of birth control pills involved millions of women. They could not have been performed if each involved person had been required to sign a separate consent form.

Appropriate safeguards against breach of confidentiality and control over medical records are essential to assure that no unauthorized person sees records and no identifying information is ever published. But, in some cases, these measures have extended to the point where research on the effects of environmental factors on health is impossible to conduct. Kenneth Rothman, a noted epidemiologist from Harvard, recently published an editorial in the *New England Journal of Medicine* in which he predicted the decline of this science over the next twenty years, ironically corresponding with its rapidly evolving sophistication and capacity to identify prime factors in preserving and protecting public health.[1]

It is difficult for a legislator faced with a bill for the protection of human subjects to ask the right questions and determine whether or not the bill is, in fact, in the public interest. To be opposed to the protection of human subjects, or to even appear to be so opposed, is politically dangerous. Yet it is a fatal error to fail to recognize that as citizens we have obligations to society that correspond to and complement society's obligations to us. In this complex age, it ought to seem obvious that the use of anonymous information gleaned from medical records and from adequately informed volunteers in medical research studies is critical to our general well-being. Without them, we are left with testimonials and trends, poor substitutions for intelligent decision-making.

"SCIENTIFIC" OBSTACLES TO HEALTH POLICY FORMATION

One of the major difficulties in translating epidemiologic research findings into reasonable health policies is the reluctance of the medical profession itself to understand the nature of this type of research. Practicing physicians are not trained in the use or understanding of numbers and statistics. They respond more readily to laboratory experiments on small numbers of subjects, where the results can be directly observed. But the kinds of issues we are discussing here cannot be observed in the laboratory. A distinguished epidemiologist and physician, Milton Terris, recently discussed the matter of evidence in an excellent article about using epidemiology as a guide to forming health policy:

> One of the major obstacles to the acceptance of epidemiological findings by clinicians relates to the character of the evidence. . . . In the middle of the nineteenth century, John Snow came to remarkably accurate conclusions on the etiology and prevention of cholera by the use of "merely statistical" evidence (which is the layman's and clinician's term of disparagement of epidemiology, i.e., the study of disease in human population groups); only later was there confirmation by so-called real science, i.e., the study of disease in rats, mice, and guinea pigs. Snow's natural experiment in the real world of London had to be validated more than a quarter of a century later by contrived experiments in the laboratory.

And so it is today. Epidemiologists have come to remarkably accurate conclusions on the etiology and prevention of a host of diseases, such as lung cancer, ischemic heart disease, and cerebrovascular disease, long before the laboratory scientists will succeed in discovering the precise pathophysiologic mechanisms that are involved. Because, as in John Snow's time, the latter information is not yet available, epidemiologists have difficulty in obtaining acceptance of their scientific conclusions and recommendations for preventive action. The lung cancer controversy is perhaps the most dramatic example of the struggles that epidemiologists have had to wage in order to overcome this obstacle.[2]

If the protection of individual members of society from risks of illnesses arising from the environment is a goal at all worth pursuing, then the careful conduct of epidemiologic studies, and their proper interpretation and use by society, are essential to the realization of that goal. We used to have infant mortality rates in excess of 40 percent of live births. We used to have life expectancies less than forty years. It is the acceptance of the need for population-based studies and the knowledge learned from them which has largely been responsible for these changes.

Chapter 4
The Transmission and
Prevention of Illness

Alternative Ways of Skinning a Cat

The great secret, known to internists and learned early in marriage by internists' wives, but still hidden from the general public, is that most things get better by themselves. Most things, in fact, are better by morning.

—Lewis Thomas

This chapter focuses on how diseases are spread and how methods of transmission provide clues to prevention. However, before discussing its transmission, it is essential to define disease. It is not generally appreciated that the definition of illness is quite arbitrary. In some societies, schizophrenics are regarded as godlike, in others as manifestations of demons. In the United States they are generally stigmatized by having the diagnosis follow them through life, preventing meaningful employment or advancement long after recovery. In China, the schizophrenic is returned to work as soon as possible and little is made of his or her absence. Thus, in different cultures, the degree of disability, and even the notion that schizophrenia is a bad thing or an illness, varies substantially.

The World Health Organization defines disease as an impairment of mental, physical, or social well-being, and I subscribe to this definition. Although this book discusses illness primarily in terms of physical impairments, it is important to bear in mind that this is because we have been so negligent in determining the causes and cures of mental and social ills that we hardly know enough to make meaningful examples of them.

DEFINING CAUSE

Most of us were introduced to the complexities of cause and effect in high school history classes when we discussed the "causes" of various wars. In my own experience, these causes were divided into immediate causes (e.g., World War I started as a result of the assassination of the Archduke Ferdinand) and underlying causes (underlying causes were always disturbingly vague and complex and seemed to involve a lot of people who misunderstood each other). Generally, I preferred the immediate causes. When asked on a test what caused World War I, I could answer a murder.

The problem arose when (and if) we got around to discussing how wars might be prevented. Would better security for the archduke have prevented that war? Obviously not. The dramatic impact of immediate causes (Pearl Harbor, the shelling of Fort Sumter, the sinking of the battleship *Maine*, and so on) often obscures the fact that the real reason wars happen is because of the complex of competing political, social, and economic issues which concern the conflicting societies.

This analogy is particularly apt in discussing disease. Ask a doctor what causes tuberculosis and chances are he will tell you that it is caused by a small bacterium, *Mycobacterium tuberculosum*, which can be spread from person to person by sputum coughed up from infected lungs. The physician is correct in the sense that without the bacteria no one would have tuberculosis, but completely wrong in implying that this little germ is the sole cause of the disease.

In the spring of 1980, a noted physician testified before a congressional subcommittee. He stated that the methods of epidemiology were not very effective in determining causes of illness, that investigators using such methods a hundred years ago thought that the causes of tuberculosis were poor sanitation and crowded housing. Now, he continued, we know the truth. A germ causes TB. What he neglected to note was that the major advances in combating tuberculosis occurred before there was an effective treatment for the disease, and they occurred as a result of improvements in sanitation and housing. Knowing those factors which facilitate the spread of the disease made it unnecessary to understand the specific bacteria involved. In fact, identification of the germ had little impact on the number of deaths from the condition. Thousands, even hundreds of thousands, have been cured of tuberculosis by modern drugs. But millions of persons have never gotten the disease because the means of transmission were thwarted.

John Stuart Mill defined it this way: "The cause, then, philosophically speaking, is the sum total of the conditions positive and negative taken together; the whole of the contingencies of every description, which being realized, the consequent invariably follows." This definition of cause is empirical and does not depend on an understanding of mechanism. Disease, like war, occurs as a result of a network of interacting factors that together produce pathology of some sort. An element in this network is often a germ, virus, bacterium, or fungus, but such organisms alone are never complete and sufficient to produce illness. At all times we carry within our bodies potentially lethal microorganisms. We keep them in check, and even use them beneficially. We are surrounded by such organisms in our external environment as well. Disease can be more accurately thought of as a breakdown in defenses than as the attack of any particular type of germ. If a breach of defenses occurs and a particular germ is eliminated, there will always be another (and consequently a different disease) to take its place. But if the defenses are maintained, invasion will not occur.

For our purposes, let us consider the causes of any particular disease as all those things which, if changed, would prevent the occurrence of that disease. We will need to modify this definition slightly to account for the fact that nature does not exist in "either/or's." A weak defense can withstand a weak assault, but not a strong one. Therefore, a given "cause" of illness may only be causative when it is sufficiently powerful to overcome whatever defenses there are against it.

THE CHAIN OF TRANSMISSION

The following story is an excellent illustration of the principles of disease transmission:

> A man had to go on a long business trip. He left his wife and home in the care of his faithful servant and left for a remote area. After several months, he returned to a city, whereupon he placed a call to his servant.
>
> "How is everything?" he asked the servant.
>
> "Fine," replied the trusted employee. "Everything is just fine, except the cat died."
>
> "The cat died!" exclaimed the man. "What happened to him?"
>
> "Well," came the answer, "he was kicked by the horse when it ran out of the barn."
>
> "How did the horse get out of the barn?"
>
> "The wall fell down," answered the servant.
>
> "What made the wall fall down?" asked the man, puzzled, for his barn had been well built.
>
> "The fire," replied his man.
>
> "What fire?"
>
> "The barn burned down," said the servant.
>
> "How did the barn catch fire?" asked the man, shocked.
>
> "From the house."

"My God," said the man, "how did the house catch fire?"
"From the curtains."
"And how did the curtains catch fire?"
"From the oil lamps in the bedroom."
"What were oil lamps doing in the bedroom?" the man asked, since their bedroom was fully electric.
"We put them there for the funeral," said the servant.
"Whose funeral?" gasped the man.
"Your wife's," said the servant.

The story can be expanded indefinitely. The point is that every event is a product of earlier events. When illness strikes, it is the product of a set, or chain, of circumstances. Preventing disease and maintaining health demands an understanding of those circumstances and intervening at the critical place in the chain.

Infectious diseases provide the clearest model for disease transmission. The successful spread of infectious disease in humans requires at least seven different factors:

1. An agent which can infect humans. This may be a virus, a bacterium, a fungus, or any of a number of less well-known microorganisms. For noninfectious diseases, the agent may be chemical (e.g., arsenic), electromagnetic (e.g., X-rays), phychologic (e.g., stress), social (e.g., poverty), or physical (e.g., accident).

2. Sufficient numbers of the agent. A minimal dose of infectious agent is required to set up an infection. This minimum dose may be quite small for some conditions, such as chicken pox (probably the most highly infectious disease known to man), or quite large for conditions such as leprosy (probably the least contagious of the infectious diseases).

3. A source of infection. An infected host or a natural reservoir of the agent must exist somewhere. This might be a contaminated water supply, spoiled food, or any of thousands of other potential sources of infection. The sources tend to be fairly specific for different types of germs. Cholera and typhoid

fever are often spread by contaminated water, for example, while Legionnaire's disease appears to spread through contaminated air conditioning equipment.

4. A suitable means of transmission. Infectious organisms have to get from place to place in order to find new hosts. Respiratory diseases have a relatively simple and direct means to this end. A cough or sneeze may spray millions of the germs into the air for others to inhale. Other germs have elaborate means for transportation. The single-celled parasites which cause malaria, for example, must be sucked up from the blood of infected individuals by specific types of mosquitos. They multiply in the mosquito and are delivered to a new host when the insect bites another person. All germs have clear and identifiable means of dispersal.

5. An entry point into a new host. There are many ways for infectious agents to enter new hosts. Respiratory viruses, for example, are usually inhaled. Malaria parasites are injected. Cholera bacilli are ingested. The tiny larvae of the parasitic disease called schistosomiasis live in water and burrow through the skin of swimmers quickly and painlessly.

6. An exit point from the host. The germ has to get out of a host in order to infect others. Many agents exit through the bowel in fecal material. The World Health Organization estimated in the 1960s that 90 percent of the world's illness could be eradicated if everyone used sanitary toilets. Other exit points are clear from the examples listed above. One of the more bizarre exit mechanisms developed by infectious agents is that of the lethal neurologic disease, kuru. This condition existed only in certain tribes in New Guinea. These people regularly consumed parts of their dead, including the brain, in order to obtain some of their characteristics. The virus was spread apparently solely through the consumption of infected human brains.

7. A susceptible host. Assuming normal health, all the measles virus around is not sufficient to induce an infection in someone who has had measles. Immunization confers resistance of

varying strength and lengths of time to diseases. Susceptibility to an illness to which we have not previously been exposed also varies according to the condition of the body's immune system.

The important thing to remember about these seven factors is that they do indeed form a chain, and a chain is only as strong as its weakest link. The essence of preventing disease is to find that weakest link and break it. We don't concern ourselves about the other six factors—unless some of them are also "breakable."

Until this century, infectious diseases were far and away the leading cause of death in the Western world. Now, however, they are relatively rare as killers, and usually, when they are fatal, they strike those whose immune systems are compromised in some way, either from age, severe physical disability, and/or as a result of medical therapies which, in the process of treating disease, also damage the immune system.

The dramatic change from infectious to noninfectious diseases as causes of death is not due primarily to improvements in medical practice, although these have certainly had an impact. In general, we do not die of those diseases which used to kill with such regularity because we are not exposed to them. In some parts of the world, 40 percent or more of the children do not celebrate a first birthday. Sanitation has led to the very modern expectation that every child born will grow to adulthood. There are no cholera or typhoid bacilli in the water we drink, no tapeworms in the meat we buy, no amoebae on the lettuce we use for salads. The food at restaurants and in the supermarkets is usually not a source of *salmonella* or *staphylococci*. Tuberculosis is uncommon principally because we no longer live in crowded, poorly ventilated homes, surviving on inadequate diets which reduce resistance to disease. Improvements in medical care have been frosting on the cake—dramatic, impressive, but only marginally contributing to the disappearance of the major causes of premature death.

The effectiveness of preventive measures is best illustrated by smallpox. As recently as 1965 more than one million people died of this disease each year. There is still *no effective treatment* for this disease, yet, in the short space of ten years, it was completely eradicated from the face of the earth (except in certain laboratories where stocks of the virus are maintained for somewhat obscure reasons). The control of smallpox required two interventions in the seven links of transmission. First, new cases were immediately isolated (block transmission) and, second, all persons who had recent contact or who lived near new cases were immediately immunized (eliminate susceptible hosts).

The smallpox virus was suited to control in these ways for several reasons. First, it occurs only in humans. Many diseases, such as yellow fever, influenza, rabies, and plague, also exist in wild animal populations from which they can be reintroduced into humans. Second, cases are not infectious until obvious skin lesions have already developed, thus permitting effective isolation before others have been infected. Most conditions become infectious before symptoms develop. Third, an effective, inexpensive, easily administered vaccine was available. Few other diseases meet all these criteria.

METHODS OF DISEASE TRANSMISSION

To interrupt the spread of disease requires an intimate understanding of the specific transmission techniques. These methods range from simple to highly complex, and a somewhat confusing nomenclature has been developed to describe the different mechanisms involved.

Essentially, the transmission of a disease is either direct, from one person directly to another, or indirect, requiring something to carry the contagious material from one person to another. Those things which carry disease material are called "vehicles" if they are inanimate. Thus, contaminated water is a vehicle for typhoid fever bacilli. Living organisms that carry disease from one person to another are called "vectors." Vectors may be mechanical, i.e., they simply carry infective material from one place to another physically, without directly participating in the growth and reproduction of that material, or they may be biologic, i.e., essential to the reproductive cycle of the infective material. House flies, for example, may serve as mechanical vectors for many diseases if they walk on fecal material, pick up germs, then fly to some foodstuffs and leave the germs on the previously uncontaminated food. Mosquitoes, on the other hand, serve as biologic vectors for malaria parasites, which must inhabit the mosquito's body during a portion of its normal life cycle. These facts are summarized in figure 4.1.

All disease occurs as a result of the interaction between an agent which produces the disease, a host in which the disease develops, and an environment which must be conducive to the development of the disease. This applies to noninfectious diseases as well as to infectious diseases. Infectious diseases have become relatively well controlled in the developed world because of the understanding we have about the means of transmission and the various ways to interrupt it. Table 4.1 lists a few communicable diseases, their principal means of spread, and the techniques used to interrupt that process.

A complete listing of the methods of transmission and control of infectious diseases is available in paperback from the American Public Health Association.[1] A glance through this book reveals four general types of infectious diseases: (1) diseases which are recognizable and common, but which are not usually very serious (e.g., mumps, chicken pox, influenza); (2) diseases which are familiar, but are less common than the first type (e.g., syphilis, hepatitis, tuberculosis); (3) diseases that are unfamiliar because they do not occur commonly in developed nations—often simply because those countries are fortunate enough not to have the required intermediate biological vectors

FIGURE 4.1
**Methods for Transmitting Disease from
One Host to Another**

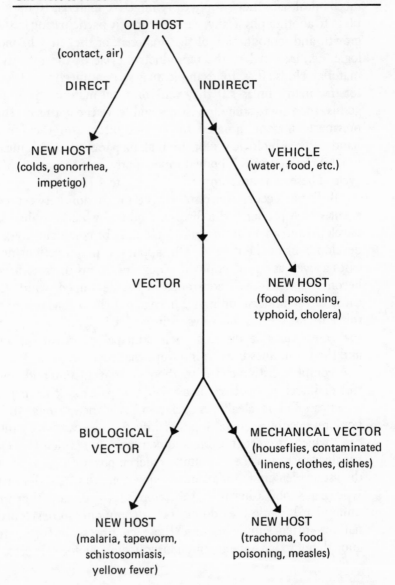

TABLE 4.1
Some Communicable Diseases and Their
Usual Means of Transmission and Control

Disease	Transmission	Control
1. Amoebic dysentery	Fecally contaminated water and vegetables, soiled hands	Sanitary feces disposal, appropriate construction and filtration of water systems, good personal hygiene
2. Cholera	As for amoebic dysentery	As for amoebic dysentery, also chlorination of water
3. Acute bacterial conjunctivitis (eye infection)	Contact with eye and respiratory discharges of infected person, direct or indirect	Personal hygiene, hygienic care of infected eyes
4. Pinworms	Direct transfer of eggs in feces to mouth or from contaminated clothes, food, occasionally by inhalation	Good personal hygiene, frequent bathing, clothing change, uncrowded housing, treatment of cases
5. Influenza	Direct contact, inhalation of respiratory particles, soiled articles of clothing	Immunization, good hygiene, quarantine
6. Malaria	Bite from infected mosquito	Control mosquito population
7. Plague	Bite of infected flea from a wild animal, especially rats; direct contact with infected person with lung involvement or open sores	Control rat population, study other wild animal populations and control those infected, isolation of patients

or because those vectors have been adequately controlled (e.g., malaria, schistosomiasis, onchocerciasis, filariasis); (4) diseases which are unfamiliar because they usually occur in wild animals and are only occasionally transmitted to man (e.g., plague, anthrax, rabies, brucellosis, tularemia). Like any classification system, some conditions remain that do not fit into any of the categories. For the moment, I classify these as miscellaneous diseases.

Of the ten leading causes of death in the United States, only pneumonia and influenza (grouped together in table 4.2) are

TABLE 4.2
Age-adjusted Death Rates per 100,000 Persons for
Ten Leading Causes of Death in the United States in 1975

Condition	Death Rate 100,000
1. Diseases of the heart	220.5
2. Malignant neoplasm (cancer)	130.9
3. Cerebrovascular diseases (stroke)	54.5
4. Accidents	44.8
5. Influenza and pneumonia	16.6
6. Cirrhosis of the liver	13.8
7. Suicide	12.6
8. Certain grouped causes of early infant mortality	12.5
9. Diabetes mellitus	11.6
10. Arteriosclerosis	6.6

SOURCE: Adapted from U.S. Department of Health, Education and Welfare, Health Resources Administration, *Health Status of Minorities and Low-Income Groups*. DHEW Publication No. (HRA) 79-627, 1979.

infectious. Although many people die of these conditions, they are usually serious in persons already debilitated by age and/or some other chronic illness. The therapy for many serious chronic illnesses frequently depresses the body's resistance to outside infection, resulting in overwhelming and fatal pneumonia or influenza. Thus, in a sense, the fact that even these conditions rank among the top ten causes of death is misleading, since they often occur as a byproduct of chronic disease.

CHRONIC (NONINFECTIOUS) DISEASE TRANSMISSION AND CONTROL

The model we have been discussing for transmission of infectious illness can be applied to chronic diseases, although the terms used have to be modified for special cases. The ten leading causes of death in the United States are listed in table 4.2. Diseases of the heart are by far the leading cause of death (about 38 percent), with cancer a distant second (about 17 percent). Cerebrovascular diseases, mostly strokes, are third on the list, and these affect mostly older persons. Over the past thirty years, an enormous effort has been made to define the causes for our high rates of these conditions, and a number of interesting, if confusing, facts have emerged.

Cigarette smoking is strongly related to the occurrence of heart disease in some countries but not in others. The level of blood cholesterol is consistently related to risk of dying from heart disease, but the relation between diet and blood cholesterol appears to be somewhat less consistent. In general, those groups consuming high levels of saturated fat (fats which are solid at room temperature, such as meat fats, solid shortenings, etc.) have more heart disease than those groups which do not. Americans have very high, but slowly declining, rates of heart disease and low rates of stroke. Japanese have low rates of heart disease, but very high rates of stroke. However, when Japanese persons immigrate to the United States, they gradually assume American rates of heart disease and stroke, suggesting that the environment plays a strong role in both conditions. The difficulties in forming a coherent picture are illustrated in figure 6.2, which lists a large sampling of factors thought to be potential causes of heart disease.

For cancer the picture is even cloudier. Cancer is not a single disease, but rather a process by which cells lose normal controls over growth and reproduction and literally consume the rest of the body in their unchecked reproduction. There are hereditary cancers, cancers caused by radiation, cancers produced by various chemicals, and cancers caused by viruses. Stomach cancer has been declining in the United States for forty years and is rare here today. In Chile and Japan, however, it is one of the most common forms of cancer, and its incidence is increasing. Cervical cancer has been declining since the 1930s, long before the introduction of the Pap smear to detect it. Esophageal cancer is rare in most parts of the world, but in one section of China it is epidemic. What is not clear for cancer or for heart disease are the patterns of interaction between the various conditions of agent, host, and environment which are required to establish the disease process and the best means for intervention.

Interestingly, the patterns of occurrence of accidents and suicide follow closely those of other causes of death in terms of predictability. This seems to emphasize the relative importance that behavioral factors play in determining susceptibility to all diseases. Hygiene, for example, is critical to protection from many infectious conditions; diet is a factor in many chronic conditions. Hygiene and diet are both related to such demographic factors as income, education, family interrelationships, and so on. These factors are also clearly related to accidents, and suicide, conditions which we normally consider separately from "health" problems. Yet note that accidents (mostly auto) and suicides rank fourth and seventh, respectively, among the ten leading causes of death. In chapter 9, I discuss in some detail the implications of the fact that accidents are the leading cause of "years of life lost." That is, if the number of deaths is multiplied by the number of years lost from a normal life expectancy, accidents are the single most serious health problem we have. This is because most persons who die in accidents are young and lose a great many years of expected life when they die.

Is it possible to apply the methods of disease prevention

which worked so well for infectious diseases to these major noninfectious killers? The answer is definitely yes, but there are two major stumbling blocks. First, susceptibility to disease increases with age. Preventing one condition in an old person simply leaves that individual vulnerable to another of the illnesses of old age. Some progress is possible with the diseases of old age, but until we develop some means for slowing the aging process, the best hope for improvements in health status certainly lies in trying to prevent premature death, that is, deaths in persons under seventy years of age. Second, much of the potential for reducing noninfectious diseases depends on personal behavior change. Infectious diseases could be approached from a societal standpoint. A government could decide to clean up the water supply, inspect restaurants and food processing companies, spray for mosquitos, and so on, which would be effective without any change in the behavior of its individual citizens. Reducing the toll from heart disease, stroke, cancer, and accidents, on the other hand, may require personal change, something that is difficult to achieve.

Table 4.3 is a partial list of noninfectious chronic diseases, factors known to be or thought to be related to transmission, and methods of intervention. The table is by no means complete with respect to mechanisms of transmission or prevention. Heredity, for example, is omitted because there is not much one can do about it. Essentially, the preventive measures boil down to those things we know we ought to do but somehow can't seem to get around to doing.

Why is that? Why do we avoid things or do things which we know are unhealthy? A very popular sign hangs in thousands of roadside cafes around the country. It says: "Everything I like is either illegal, immoral, or fattening." The implication is that whatever is good for you isn't much fun. Yet, a moment's thought proves that is not true. There are runners who are enthusiastic to the point of fanaticism about their running, vegetarians who genuinely do not like meat, people who simply

TABLE 4.3
Some Noninfectious Chronic Diseases and
Means of Their "Transmission" and Control

Disease	Transmission	Control
1. Heart disease	High fat diet; lack of exercise; high blood pressure; cigarette smoking; stress	Low fat diet; exercise; control of blood pressure; not smoking; relaxation; stress reduction
2. Cancer	Radiation; chemicals; smoking; viruses (?); diet	Reduce radiation exposure (less sun, X-rays only when necessary, etc.); avoid exposure to carcinogenic chemicals; not smoking; low-fat high-fiber diet
3. Cerebrovascular disease	High blood pressure; smoking; high fat diet (?)	Control blood pressure; not smoking; low-fat diet
4. Accidents	Not using seat belts; speeding; poisons improperly secured; unsafe equipment; intoxication	Use of seat belts; secure toxic chemicals; safe design; maintenance of equipment; not using mechanical equipment while intoxicated; alcoholism prevention or treatment
5. Cirrhosis of liver	Alcoholism	Alcoholism prevention or treatment

don't feel right without a seat belt around them in a car, non-smokers who are positively nauseated by cigarettes, meditators for whom stress control through relaxation and meditation are essential concomitants to an enjoyable life, drinkers who never want to get drunk, and so on. Enjoyment, like beauty, is always in the eye of the beholder. A prime rib roast, steaming hot and oozing fat onto a puffy Yorkshire pudding, is not an appealing sight to a vegetarian. Before we can interrupt the transmission of chronic diseases, we must examine and understand why two persons can react so differently to the same stimulus. It brings us into the realms of sociology, behavioral sciences, economics, and politics—all of which are intimately tied to our health behaviors and, consequently, to our health status and risk of dying from various diseases. If the government subsidizes the sale of carcinogens, as it does with tobacco price supports, the government itself becomes a contributor to the second-leading cause of death, and politics and economics become closely bound to our health status. Similarly, when nearly all illnesses are far more common among the poor, social programs become health issues. Certainly, the use of seat belts is one of the major health issues of our time, in view of the fact that they are the single best preventive measure against premature death in automobile accidents (the leading cause of death among persons aged fifteen to forty-five).

In 1979 the Department of Health, Education, and Welfare issued a lengthy report on health promotion and disease prevention.[2] The second chapter of this report is a brief overview of risks to good health. It states: "The importance of behavioral factors in the etiology of diverse diseases is becoming increasingly recognized by health professionals and is described in virtually all of the papers that focus on preventing specific disorders." The report proceeds to explain that poverty is one of the key correlates of ill health, and that deterioration of family ties has clear health-related effects, since as a social support system the family has an impact on an individual's capacity to resist illnesses.

Although they do not quite make the top ten causes of death, homicides are also distressingly common in our society and becoming more frequent all the time. In 1976 there were 19,554 homicides in the United States, and more than 90 percent of these were intentional and unjustifiable murders. Homicide is the *second* leading cause of death among young, black males, a group characterized by poverty, unemployment and social disorganization—all consistent correlates of homicide rates. Except in wartime, there has probably never been a nation in world history with a higher homicide rate than the United States (approximately 1 in 10,000 persons is murdered each year). Those who wish to divorce the discussion of health and social issues can never meaningfully address most of those conditions which kill and disable. The old idea that one cause leads to one disease is not tenable even for infectious conditions. For noninfectious health problems it is little short of ludicrous.

The major contributors to our commonest health problems are negative personal behaviors, unsafe workplaces, unsafe home and out-of-work environments, poverty and its attendant furies, social disruption, and bad legislation. These are strong links in the chain of cause. Breaking them will require clarity of purpose and diligence on the parts of both individuals and society as a whole.

Very little modification is required to apply the requirements for transmission of infectious disease to chronic, noninfectious conditions.

1. An agent—in this case the agent does not "infect," but rather it "affects" human beings. It may be a toxic chemical, a stressful environment, a hazardous personal behavior, radiation, and so on. Further, a given condition may have multiple agents involved, a fact which leads to some of the contradictory and confusing information discussed earlier.

2. Sufficient numbers—as with infectious disease, a sufficient amount of the agent or agents must be present to overcome the body's defenses. The amount of a carcinogenic chemical, for example, which is required to initiate a cancer may vary considerably depending on other factors in the physical, social, and psychologic environment of the individual.

3. A source—a factory, the tobacco counter, or the underlying reasons for hazardous behavior.

4. Suitable means of transmission—air and water can play this role for toxic materials. So, too, can cigarette smoke, ad-

vertising, and poor physical, social, and psychologic environment, inadequate education, economic pressures, and so on.

5. An entry point—direct as for chemical and electromagnetic agents, subtle and indirect for social, psychologic ones.

6. An exit point—a smokestack, the end of a cigarette, training of a child by one whose behaviors are unhealthy, an economic system which perpetuates unhealthy behaviors by making others financially dependent on repeating the unhealthy activities which support that system.

7. A susceptible host—this also applies to biologic, social and psychologic susceptibility. Resistance is highly variable, but far from unlimited.

In general, each specific illness has immediate and general causes, and quickest results are seen when immediate causes are eradicated. But, returning to the analogy that opened this chapter, elimination of the immediate cause of a war will probably only delay the action, not forestall it. Particularly for chronic conditions, the impact of changing underlying causes such as diet, stress, exercise, etc. may require long periods of time. But those effects will be far-reaching and not limited to a single disease type. In essence, understanding factors which produce and support a condition of less than optimal health can lead to a coordinated effort by the individual and by society to create an environment which is healthier.

In the meantime, while you are waiting for society to come along and do its part, you personally can sever a number of the links by making changes in personal behavior that are simple, direct, and for the most part limited to the things suggested in table 4.3.

Chapter 5
Finding the Causes

Why Things Are Never as Simple as They Seem

There is no objective scientific way of making decisions, nor is it likely that there ever will be.

—National Academy of Sciences

"What?" people say to me when I quote the above statement. "No objective way of making decisions? Why, science, when properly performed, is the essence of objectivity. It is the only way to eliminate human bias in the decision-making process."

It is amazing how many people are sensitive about this subject. It seems we all have a stake in a belief that there is one "true" means for pursuing truth. I confess to a certain fondness for making outrageous statements. They prod people into examining closely held assumptions. At the same time we are reacting, somewhere deep underneath we are asking ourselves, "Why am I reacting so strongly to this? Perhaps I *am* dogmatic on the subject."

Human beings develop fervent beliefs in response to at least two motivations: (1) we believe as we have been taught and (2) we believe what it is in our own self-interest to believe. When these come into conflict with each other, we usually choose self-interest over teaching.

This explains why opposing sides in any "scientific" argument can always produce experts to support their views. The tobacco companies can find a physician who doesn't believe cigarettes cause disease. The dairy industry has nutritionists who believe that it doesn't matter how much fat is in your diet so long as it comes from milk, cream, butter, and cheese. Nutritionists for the National Livestock and Meat Board believe that pork and beef fat are beneficial. American Heart Association nutritionists, on the other hand, will turn pale at the sight of a hot fudge sundae or a slab of bacon. All of these people are well trained, dedicated, and sincere people. They have selectively evaluated available information in order to arrive at a conclusion which is in their self-interest to hold. Each of us makes similar choices in similar ways. When general belief patterns do change, it is often because the weight of evidence for a particular idea leans so preponderantly in one direction that it becomes difficult to persist in an alternative idea unless one is willing to forego all evidence and accept the idea on faith alone. That, too, occurs.

MAKING HEALTH DECISIONS

How, then, is it possible to make sense out of the huge amounts of health information we have? Understanding health, or any other controversial subject, hinges on observing these basic ideas:

1. Know the limitations of information about health. No single study or book or paper ever proved anything. Seek confirmation.

2. Understand the nature of the various types of studies and their relative reliability. Some studies are designed to seek hy-

potheses, not to finally answer questions. The media are usually not aware of this distinction. Your doctor may not be either. Some studies are simply inadequate and should never have been done.

3. Take every author's interpretation of his study findings with a grain of salt. Where possible, look at the findings themselves and ask yourself if your conclusions are the same.

4. Strike a balance between staying open to new ideas and rejecting those not based on evidence. Some ideas persist because strong evidence supports them. Others persist despite substantial evidence against them. Still others have never been adequately examined and might be valid. There are many practices performed by alternative health practitioners, such as naturopaths, chiropractors, acupuncturists, and other health specialists that have simply not received adequate scientific testing to make firm conclusions as to their efficacy. Often, they have not had such testing because of the resistance of the medical establishment to providing the resources it controls for the purpose of such testing. In the same way that much of standard medical practice is useful and much is not, it is likely that the therapies of other health traditions have mixed efficacy. After all, each of these paths is followed by many reasonable and intelligent people. One significant health problem is the antipathy among different sorts of practitioners. A marriage of disciplines and formal testing of everyone's sacred cows would benefit all.

This chapter focuses principally on the second item, understanding different types of studies. Chapter 6 deals with simple techniques for judging the quality of information.

TYPES OF STUDIES AND WHAT CAN BE LEARNED FROM EACH

1. The experiment. There are many different kinds of scientific studies. The most obvious and best known is the experimental study, in which conditions are carefully controlled by

the experimenter, to the best of his or her ability. The only variation between two groups that are compared is the single factor being studied. In some fields, the degree of control over outside, or distorting, variability has even resulted in the breeding of strains of genetically identical test animals. Experimental studies can never, in the classical sense, be performed on human beings. Techniques which approximate experiments are used, such as the intervention trial discussed below, but there are no true experiments on humans because of ethical constraints and the impossibility of holding all conditions constant. One can *decide* what a mouse will eat, but only *recommend* what a human will eat. This is a critical distinction. Many commercial interests reject all animal studies which suggest that their products may have adverse health effects in humans because animals are not, after all, people and experiments in the classical sense have not been performed on humans. In their self-righteous denial of evidence they neglect to note that such studies cannot be performed with humans and that decisions about safety must be reached using the imperfect approaches discussed below.

2. The survey. America is the land of surveys. Television programs live or die according to the results of surveys. Elections get decided, at least in part, by the survey results published in the media on a monotonously regular basis. Sometimes they're right, sometimes not. We all seem to like keeping score, even if we view the results with a jaundiced eye. This survey mania is an unfortunate development in modern society. In the first place, a survey is at best only a "photograph" of a current situation. Unless repeated frequently, surveys cannot show the dynamics of any situation. To be valid, surveys must be conducted under very rigid and specific conditions such that the results are truly representative of the population to which they are applied. The poll which predicted a landslide victory by Dewey over Truman is a classic example of a nonrepresentative survey. The poll was conducted by telephone, but in 1948 a substantial number of poorer Americans did not have telephones. Thus, the

survey seriously undercounted lower-income voters who strongly favored Truman. With respect to health issues, surveys are principally useful in assessing current health practices and ideas and measuring the prevalence of disease in the population.

Table 5.1 presents the major types of studies discussed here with their principal uses. The prevalence of a disease is the

TABLE 5.1
Principal Types of Studies on the Causes and Prevention of Disease

Type of Study	Rela- tive Cost	Dura- tion	Show Cause?	Comments
1. Experiment	Low	Short (usually)	Yes	Seldom feasible in humans
2. Survey	Low	Short	No	Assess current situation
3. Case-control study	Low	Short	No	Find "risk factors" associated with health and illness
4. Prospective	High	Long	No	Determine relationship over time between risk factor and disease
5. Intervention study	Very high	Long	Yes	Seldom feasible because of high cost and time required

actual rate of a disease in a population, the number of cases present at a given point in time divided by the number of persons in the population. Prevalence also depends on both the incidence (number of new cases per unit time) and the duration of each individual case. Thus, if the death rate for a disease rises while the incidence remains constant, the prevalence will *decrease* because the victims are dying more quickly. Major influenza epidemics are followed by a decrease in prevalence of chronic respiratory diseases, because people with these conditions are especially likely to die from an influenza infection.

Prevalence will also decrease if the incidence decreases or if a new medical treatment shortens the course of a disease. Actual prevalence levels in a population are a result of all of these factors working together.

Prevalence levels may also be affected by a change in the definition of a disease. Every ten years the World Health Organization issues a revision of the International Classification of Diseases. Changes in the way a condition is defined may lead to substantial differences in prevalence rates.

Surveys are a means for setting health priorities and identifying areas of change within the population only when those who are surveyed are truly representative of the group to which the results are referred. This cannot be overemphasized. Remember, surveys must be representative, and they determine only prevalence, never cause.

3. The case-control study. This is the standard means for developing hypotheses about the causes of a disease. It is also one of the least expensive types of study to conduct and, as a consequence, case-control studies are widely, and often improperly, performed. The method is simple. Identify a group of persons who have a given disease, then another group with whom to compare them. Ask lots of questions, do lots of tests, then determine which of the questions and tests are associated with one of the groups more than the other. Statistical tests have been designed to determine the "significance" of these relationships. That is, they assess whether or not the occurrence of a given factor in association with disease (or nondisease) is likely to be due to chance alone. These tests do *not* measure the importance of the factor in determining disease. They say nothing about whether or not the relationship is causal, that is, they do not indicate that the disease is caused by the factor.

For example, suppose you want to study the causes of cervical cancer and that, prior to your study, nothing was known about the factors that contribute to this disease. As a first step, you obtain a list of cervical cancer cases from the local tumor registry. With most diseases there are no convenient registries that permit easy identification of cases, but in this instance you are lucky. Next, you decide to randomly select a number of persons from the city directory to compare with the cases. You use all the proper techniques to insure that this is a representative "control" group. Now, you do a careful interview with each case and each control to determine how they differ. The first thing you discover is that cervical cancer is strongly associated with sex. Only females get it. So what, you say, I knew that. Let's get on with it and look at some other factors. Right away you are in trouble. Since your selection of controls was truly random, half of them are males, and, therefore, not susceptible to cervical cancer. You have only half a control group left, and there simply aren't enough of them to draw any conclusions about other factors. What did you do wrong? Nothing. Sex is strongly associated with cervical cancer, and your conclusions from this first attempt reveal that. The study also shows you that this relationship with sex is so powerful that it can obscure other causal relationships which you are trying to identify. Therefore, in order to eliminate this bias, you must choose only women in your control group. This process is an example of stratification, and it must be performed in many studies which aren't so obvious so that powerful associations don't hide less powerful ones. If you had analyzed your original set of data, you could have drawn authentic-looking tables and figures designed to prove that there is no relationship between cervical cancer and any other factor except sex. But in your heart you would know that this was simply because, after removing the effect of sex, your sample size was not large enough to observe any other effects. A newspaper reporter, however, cannot be expected to know this, and even if he or she does, the chances are that the opportunity for a quick headline will influence his or her judgment.

So you get a new control group composed of women who fall into the same age groups as your cases. (You learned from your first mistake. Recognizing that age is strongly related to many health issues and that age differences in cases and controls might lead to some screwy conclusions, you decided to stratify by age groups as well.) You now find that women who have cervical cancer are more likely to have had multiple sex partners, to have started intercourse at an early age, to be non-Jewish, to have had early pregnancies and earlier and more marriages, to have had herpes virus sometime in the past, and to have taken oral contraceptives for longer periods of time than controls. These eight factors are significantly associated with cervical cancer.

To be a cause of a disease, a factor must be associated with that disease. But many things are associated with diseases but do not cause them. Chronic respiratory disease is associated with lack of exercise, for example, but in this case it is the disease which prevents the exercise, not the other way around. So, what happens now? You have factors associated with the disease in question. Such factors are often called "risk factors" because when they are present disease is more likely to also be present. This does *not* mean that everyone who has one or more of these factors will get cervical cancer, nor does it mean that any of the factors *cause* disease. In fact, as noted above, some risk factors might even result from the disease in question.

The important thing to recognize is that case-control studies can't really take us very much further. Where the association is overwhelming and also fits preconceived notions of cause and effect, we might interpret the results as causal with some degree of confidence, but never with certainty. The case-control study cannot tell you which came first, the factor or the disease, and it cannot tell you if modification of the factor could prevent the disease. Other types of studies are required to do these things.

4. The prospective or longitudinal study. Prospective studies permit the determination of the proper time sequence between risk factor and disease. Because they require disease-free persons and measure the occurrence of illness in a group over time, such studies are expensive and time-consuming. When examined

within a time frame that is reasonable for scientific investigators, nearly all diseases are rare. Dental caries and common colds may be exceptions, but most other conditions occur infrequently during a period of one to five years. In a prospective study, the effective size of the study population is the number of persons who become diseased during the observation period, rather than the total number of participating individuals. Thus, prospective studies often involve many thousands of persons. The Framingham study, for example, is one of the most important epidemiologic studies of the modern era. More than five thousand healthy persons have been regularly examined over three decades in order to determine the early clues to later illness. Such studies can determine which factors precede illness and significantly predict future occurrences of various illnesses. They cannot, however, prove cause. They can be used to select factors most likely to lead to a reduction in illness for use in intervention studies.

5.   The cohort study. This type of study is actually a special case of the prospective study. A cohort is a single group of individuals followed over time. Cohorts are useful in examining theories of health and disease for identifying effects due to changes in society through time. For example, if a survey reveals that 20 percent of males over age sixty-five have high blood pressure, we might wonder if men just naturally get high blood pressure as they age or if this is due to other outside factors. One way to answer this question is to compare past surveys for men in the same age group. A 1940 survey of men aged sixty-five to seventy contains those born between 1870 and 1875. A 1950 survey of men aged sixty-five to seventy contains those born between 1880 and 1885, a 1960 survey has those born between 1890 and 1895, and a 1970 survey includes those born between 1900 and 1905. At the time of measurement each group was the same age, but their birth years are different. If the same proportion of these men have high blood pressure on each survey we might conclude that this is a normal effect of aging. If the proportions

differ, then we might conclude that there is some environmental cause for the change. Each separate birth period (e.g., 1870 to 1875) is called a birth cohort.

6. The intervention study. The closest thing to proof of cause in humans arises from intervention studies. These are also prospective in design. However, in addition to beginning with healthy people and following them over time to determine which diseases they eventually develop, a portion of the group also receives an intervention program designed to reduce whatever risk factor is being examined. An intervention study was done by the Veterans Administration in the 1960s to determine if treating mild high blood pressure with drugs would reduce the frequency of deaths in the treated group compared to those who were not treated. (At the time, almost no one received treatment for mild hypertension, so the trial was quite ethical. It could not be repeated today because of the knowledge that it generated.) This required a large group of persons with high blood pressure. Some were treated actively, others received placebos. Over a period of several years, it became obvious that those receiving active treatment had lower death rates.

An intervention trial which tested the effect of cigarettes on lung cancer, though, would be unfeasible. The lag time between smoking and lung cancer probably exceeds twenty years. The rate of the disease, even among smokers, is relatively low. Consequently, the costs of such a study would be prohibitive. For the same reason, no one has performed a longitudinal intervention study of the effectiveness of reducing intake of fat and cholesterol in lowering the rates of heart attack. With respect to many such issues policies must be formulated using inadequate kinds of information. Where information is not definitive, the consistency of results from study to study (at least those that are well designed) and the congruence of that information to studies on animals and laboratory investigations must be relied on in making intelligent personal decisions and developing public policy.

OBSERVATION VERSUS
CLINICAL TRIALS

Another way to view human studies is to divide them into those requiring only observation and those which necessitate direct involvement in the treatment or behavior of the participants. The second type is usually termed a "clinical trial." Intervention studies are a kind of clinical trial, as are direct human studies of therapeutic measures. By law, new drugs must have clinical trials before they may be licensed and prescribed, although such studies cannot be large enough to detect rare or long-term side effects because of the prohibitive costs associated with finding such effects. Birth control pills, for example, were used by millions of women for many years before their association with an increased risk of heart attack and stroke was detected.

Whatever our qualms about the ethics of clinical trials involving human beings, it is clear that it is even more unethical not to conduct such trials:

> The ethical justification for such experimentation, which is outside the pure physician-patient relationship, is based on a judgment that in certain circumstances it is legitimate to put a subject at risk, with his or her consent, because of the overriding need of society for progress in combating certain diseases.[1]

Medical practices, unlike new drugs, need not be subjected to clinical trials prior to general implementation. The many practices discussed in chapter 8 are examples of the problems created by this lack of testing. The same applies to practices designed to maintain health. A trip to any bookstore will amply supply the unwary buyer with hundreds of sure cures and methods for achieving and maintaining optimal health. Many contradict each other, despite the dogmatic assertions by their authors that their approach is the way to positive health. Do you follow Dr. Atkins' high fat diet to lose weight when the American Heart

Association views it as downright dangerous? Should you take vitamin E? High doses of vitamin C? Become a vegetarian? Eat lots of red meat? Fast? Get rolfed? Go into any of several dozen therapies? Eat only organic foods? Exercise? Drink more alcohol? Less alcohol?

This list of real recommendations could probably be extended for several pages. For a few of the practices (e.g., exercise, low-fat diet, not smoking, reducing stress) there is suggestive data indicating that they are beneficial. Most of the rest are simply untested. They may sound great. They may fit our philosophical views of the world (or contradict them), but a meaningful answer to the question of their usefulness is simply not available.

A widely known authority who emphasizes proper diet as a means for achieving and maintaining optimal health, has responded to this confusing situation with yet another book.[2] He asks his readers to accept his version of the truth because it is corroborated by the International Society for Research on Nutrition and Diseases of Civilization as well as by the "empirical evidence of centuries and milleniums of actual application." He asks us to accept the fact that actual human experience (anecdote) is a better guide than animal tests and laboratory research. But everything we know about the selective nature of information-gathering which produces anecdotal tales of benefit tells us that this is an inappropriate means of judging benefits. Blood-letting is also based on a tradition thousands of years old and was long the single most important tool in the physician's armamentarium.

I am not taking issue with the author's ideas, many of which I personally believe are sound. Instead, I am trying to inject a note of caution. Unquestioned acceptance of a single approach, whether its source is a physician, some other authority, or the man next door, can be detrimental to the making of a good choice. Investigate. Ask questions. What kinds of studies support these ideas? Do two different approaches appear sound? Why not do both? Experiment.

The truth is that using empirical data I can prove most anything I want to. All I have to do is select my data appropriately. I could easily determine that more than 90 percent of children with colds who eat turnips are over their colds within two weeks. But to declare that turnips cure colds would be erroneous, since colds are nearly always short-lived no matter what one does. If this seems obvious, consider that in the 1950s infants with an eye disease called retrolental fibroplasia were often treated with adrenocorticotrophic hormone. Improvement occurred in 75 percent of cases with this therapy. Only later was it discovered that 75 percent of such infants improved whether they had the therapy or not.

INTERPRETING THE RESULTS OF CLINICAL TRIALS

It is certainly fair, then, to ask about the reliability of the results of clinical trials. If such studies are performed, can we have confidence in the results? Unfortunately, the answer is "not necessarily." A particularly glaring example, recently retold in the *British Medical Journal*, concerns a 1930 study in England which concluded that school children given supplemental milk gained more weight than those who did not receive the milk.[3] Three-quarters of a pint of raw milk was given daily to five thousand children. Another five thousand received the same amount of pasteurized milk. Ten thousand children received no milk and were weighed and measured as controls. The two groups that received the milk gained more weight and height during the five months of the study than those who did not receive it. But the study began in February (winter) and ended in June. Children were weighed with their clothes on. It was later determined that sympathetic teachers had selectively placed the poorer children in the milk groups. The poorer children had fewer winter clothes. So, when they were weighed in February, they weighed less. In the warmer June weather, the weight difference of the clothes of the rich and poor children was gone, so the poor looked as if they had gained more weight.

Experts in study design should be able to spot errors such as this. The public cannot. Each individual's protection from false conclusions lies in his or her own seeking of confirmation. Two studies seldom have identical sources of error or bias. With three or four studies, the chance is even less that the same flaws are shared. Seek confirmation from more than a single source.

In summary, there are many kinds of studies which examine health status and its associated causes in people. These range from simple observations of what is going on in a population to attempts to understand the factors associated with health and illness, to efforts to determine the effects of changing various associated factors as a means of determining cause and intervention strategies. The inference of cause requires knowledge, including all available types of studies and confirmatory animal and laboratory information.

Health is a product of our lives, including physical, emotional, and psychological history and state. For this reason, the identification of risk factors allows only an estimate of the odds that an event such as an illness will occur. Such predictions are highly accurate when applied to groups (e.g., a group of smokers will experience eight to ten times as many lung cancers as a similar group of nonsmokers), but cannot point to the specific individuals who will be affected. The best chance for maintaining good health comes from a careful observation of conflicting claims, a selection of those which are well founded, and action to reduce the level of risk present in each individual.

Chapter 6
Statistics and the Misuse
of Information

**Why Everything Seems
to Be Bad for Us and
What to Do about It**

*It is impossible to make
anything foolproof
because fools are so
ingenious.*

—Murphy's Eleventh Law

Michael Dalton is fifty-seven
years old and fat. He also has a
moderately elevated serum
cholesterol level, smokes thirty
cigarettes a day, and never exercises.
He used to do a considerable
amount of hiking and fishing, but
seldom goes out of doors these
days. He denies feeling unwell and
certainly is not aware of any
shortness of breath, but knows that
he couldn't possibly take the hikes
he used to take a few years back.

Mr. Dalton (not his real name)
is a participant in a nationwide
heart disease prevention research
program called the Multiple Risk
Factor Intervention Trial. A
screening program in 1974 identified him as having an exceptionally
high risk for developing heart
disease, and he was enrolled in an

aggressive program to reduce that risk. Since that time, he has gained eleven pounds, takes antihypertensive medications sporadically, smokes as much as ever, and still does not exercise. His diet, likewise, has not changed, despite the efforts by the study staff to assist him and despite his continued cooperation in attending the appointments set up for him.

Recently, Michael Dalton told me why he has made no changes. His words have a familiar ring. "What's the use?" he told me, "These days it seems like everything is bad for you. It's not worth living in a closet to reach ninety. Everything you eat causes cancer, and everything else you enjoy causes heart disease. What's the point in trying to change anything?"

I stammered a half-hearted answer about the advantages of making just a few changes and went back to my office in a thoughtful mood. I took a pen and began jotting down various factors that have been reported to cause heart disease. In five minutes I had thirty-eight items on the list, and I was chuckling. No wonder Mr. Dalton was confused, especially when one considered that many of the items were based on the loosest of information and some actually contradicted each other.

For example, from my files I found a June 1975 article from a daily San Francisco Bay area newspaper which was headlined: Heart Attacks from Lack of 'C'? The assistant professor quoted in the story had done studies on rabbits. He was quoted as saying, "I keep playing devil's advocate, asking all the questions my critics will ask. But all the pieces of the puzzle fit. It has to be right."

Next to that item was a news clipping from an August 1975 issue of the *National Enquirer*. The headline read: People Who Take Vitamin C Increase Their Chances of a Heart Attack. The "top medical researcher" quoted in this story had worked with rats and concluded that his experimental animals which "were essentially middle-aged, comparable to people in their forties and fifties" had higher cholesterol levels when fed vitamin C than did those fed similar diets without vitamin C. From this he inferred that the vitamins increased the risk of heart attack in humans. The problem with both of these stories is not that the studies were improperly performed, but rather that a single animal study had given rise to banner headlines and national publicity falsely inferring cause to either lack or excess of vitamin C.

By comparison, the relationship of increased cholesterol level to heart disease has been reconfirmed in hundreds of studies involving tens of thousands of persons all over the world. The relationship has been observed in animals. It has been noted that people who get heart disease have higher blood cholesterol on the average than those who do not. To prove that the heart disease did not itself lead to these high blood cholesterol levels, persons with high and low cholesterol have been observed over periods of up to thirty years. It has been clearly shown that those with higher cholesterol levels twenty to thirty years ago developed more heart disease as time went on than did those with lower cholesterol levels. Even this does not constitute absolute proof of cause, but it is a fairly strong circumstantial case. There is immeasurable difference in the evidence for asserting that cholesterol level is *one* of the causes of heart disease as opposed to vitamin C being *the* cause. Yet vitamin C, because it was a new "cause," grabbed the headlines.

While there are dozens of speculative ideas about factors possibly related to heart disease, there are relatively few factors that are most certainly causes of heart attacks. Mr. Dalton (and most of the rest of us) lacks a means for judging the information that he reads with respect to its validity for him. What things should he simply note with interest, and what should he *act* on?

Many people are highly distrustful of statistics. Others are completely credulous, accepting everything they read. As is usually the case, truth lies somewhere between those extremes. Your chance of being misled can be dramatically reduced if you respond to conclusions based on statistics with a set of questions about the data. Errors of statistical interpretation nearly always fall into one of five categories (table 6.1). None of these requires any training in statistics or mathematics to understand. The remainder of this chapter is devoted to describing these types of errors and learning how to recognize them.

TYPES OF STATISTICAL ERRORS

1. Conclusions based on insufficient information. In a sense, all other errors are a subtype of this one. For the purposes of this discussion, however, this type of error refers specifically to those

TABLE 6.1
**Common Statistical Errors and the Questions You Should
Ask Yourself When Evaluating Statistical Information**

Error Type	Question
1. Conclusion based on insufficient information	1. Have these conclusions been confirmed by other controlled studies?
2. Errors of comparison a. Lack of a control group	2a. Is there a control or comparison group?
b. Incorrect control group	b. Is the control group similar to the study group in all important respects?
c. Improper generalization	c. Are the results generalized to groups similar enough to the study group to justify the generalization?
3. Using the wrong statistics	3. Are these the appropriate statistics for arriving at the conclusion given?
4. Asking the unanswerable question	4. Can the information presented be accurately obtained? Were the same criteria applied to all comparison groups?
5. Misinterpretation	5. Is it possible to reach the conclusions presented from the data that was collected?

instances in which broad and sweeping conclusions are based on one or two small studies which are insufficient in size or design to warrant the grandiose conclusions.

The two articles on vitamin C and heart disease, discussed above, are examples of this common error of interpretation. Both articles assume that the "answer" to heart disease had been discovered through a single small-animal experiment. In neither case was heart disease actually studied. In the first instance, vitamin C seemed to produce a change in the biochemistry of the arterial wall which the investigator *assumed* to be beneficial. In the second, vitamin C produced a rise in the level of blood cholesterol in rats, which the investigator *assumed* would lead to a rise in heart disease. This last assumption is especially suspect, since the total blood cholesterol level is determined by adding up three different cholesterol fractions in the blood. Of these fractions, the first (very low density lipoprotein) is only weakly associated with heart disease, the second (low density lipoprotein) is strongly and positively associated with heart disease, and the third (high density lipoprotein) is strongly but *negatively* associated with heart disease. Thus, if the rise in cholesterol were due to a rise in high density lipoprotein, we might actually expect the heart disease rate to decline. Both of these studies could be accurate. The errors lie in the interpretations assigned to the results. Both cases represent preliminary work requiring confirmation and validation.

Many things have been causally linked to heart disease in the scientific and popular press. Figure 6.1 lists the thirty-eight different factors that have been associated with an increased incidence of coronary heart disease. I assembled this list after talking to Mr. Dalton. The list is by no means complete. It is no service to the public for a newspaper to pick up reports of preliminary studies, which are directed primarily at identifying hypotheses for further testing, and treat them as established findings. Even the well-informed lay person cannot look at figure 6.1 and determine from it which actions he or she could

FIGURE 6.1
Some Risk Factors for Heart Disease

Hypertension	Glucose intolerance
Cigarette smoking	Sedentary life style
Elevated serum cholesterol	Heredity
Elevated serum triglycerides	Nonspecific ECG changes
High fat diet	Xanthine oxidase (in milk)
High sugar diet	General life stress levels
Diet high in vitamin C	Diminished vital capacity
Diet low in vitamin C	Arrhythmias
Soft water	Positive exercise ECG
Geographic mobility	Male sex
Job changes	Elevated phospholipids
Marital status	Elevated uric acid
Chromium deficiency	Hypothyroidism
Cadmium	Short stature
Zinc	Abnormal balistocardiogram
Coffee	Oral contraceptives
Personality type	Inadequate social support systems
Low alpha cholesterol level	Dietary salt
Obesity	Low fiber diet

take to reduce the risk of heart disease. There is no perspective, no context in which to place the findings. The truth is that the tired old stories, the ones you hear time and time again, represent by far the most reliable approaches to preventing disease. Cholesterol and diet, for example, are still around as issues after twenty-five years, precisely because the evidence for a causal relationship is so compelling. The same is true for cigarette smoking. Controversy continues to revolve about these risk factors, mostly because there are powerful groups which have an economic interest in the status quo.

The treatment of high blood pressure, by contrast, is clearly beneficial. No economic interests bar the way to modifying treatment practices for hypertension. As a consequence, such practices have changed dramatically over the past ten years, despite the fact that the evidence favoring treatment of high blood pressure, while strong, is hardly more convincing than that suggesting that Americans should eat less fat and quit smoking.

This is not to say that the other thirty-five risk factors are irrelevant. Some, such as male sex and glucose intolerance, cannot be modified, so where they exist as risk factors they can only indicate that even more emphasis should be placed on those factors which are modifiable. Others, such as low alpha cholesterol level and coronary prone (type A) behavior, are strong predictors of heart disease. Effective means of modification are still being studied. Most of the rest represent hypotheses not yet well enough understood to warrant either individual or social action. Some, in time, may be recognized as important contributors.

A "sudden breakthrough" leading to the immediate conquest of heart disease, cancer, stroke, or other chronic diseases simply will not occur. These conditions are produced through a combination of many factors. Diet, smoking and exercise, lifestyle, and stress are all involved, as are blood pressure, heredity, and probably many other things. No single factor is going to explain or prevent the disease. Even if a one-hundred-percent effective treatment were developed for heart attack and stroke, they would remain major causes of death simply because most persons who die of these conditions die before they get to a doctor. Treatment and prevention are totally separate issues. We have, for example, a highly effective treatment for syphilis. Yet today there is more syphilis in this country than there was before penicillin was available.

A single study can never provide proof of any scientific truth. Therefore, always ask yourself, "Have these conclusions been confirmed by other controlled studies?" The importance of controlled studies and how they differ from uncontrolled ones is discussed below.

2. Errors in comparison. Suppose you are the director of the Arizona State Department of Health and you receive a report from one of your staff that the death rate from stroke in one city is twenty times higher than the stroke death rate in another city. Further, the first city's death rate is twenty-three

times the national average death rate for stroke. Do you evacu-
ate the first town? Move everyone from there to the second city?
Quit your job? Have a stroke of your own?

There are many optional responses to this situation. None of
the ones suggested so far appears to be productive, so perhaps
another approach is in order. Let's assume that you begin by
asking for a little more information. "What are the names of
the two cities?" you ask your assistant. "The first one is Sun City
and the second is Phoenix," he answers. At that point your
blood pressure drops back to normal. You hand your assistant
a copy of a basic book on epidemiology and suggest that he
read it.

Your assistant forgot two things. First, stroke is primarily a
disease of old age, and second, Sun City is a retirement town,
filled almost exclusively with elderly people. The high rate of
stroke there is a result of nothing more than the age of its resi-
dents. Although the example may seem overly simplistic, in fact,
the comparison of noncomparable groups probably constitutes
the single most common error in the medical and popular literature on health and disease.

For example, in December 1971, the San Francisco Chroni-
cle carried a news item stating that mothers who have only one
child do not live as long as mothers who have three or more
children. The story finished by saying that the reason "remains
unclear, but statistics show such is the case." Two groups are
compared—mothers with one child and mothers with three or
more children. Question: Are these two groups comparable
enough to make the comparison about life expectancy which
has been made? They are not, of course, and the difference is
critical and the claim is completely incorrect.

Mothers with three or more children are necessarily older, on
the average, than mothers with one child—since it takes more
years to have all those children. In order to be included in the
group with three or more children, a woman had to survive until she was old enough to have them. Let us say, for example,

that after the first birth a woman averages about twenty-one years of age, and after the third birth the average age of the mother is thirty-one years of age. Then, in order to be included in the second group the woman had to live to be thirty-one years old. If, on the other hand, she had a child at twenty-one, and died at twenty-three in an automobile accident she would be in the group with one child and her death would considerably shorten average life expectancy. There is no risk of death between ages twenty-one and thirty-one for women with three or more children, since they have to live to be thirty-one to be in the group. An extreme case of this might be made with the following statement: Men who live to be eighty years old are more likely to live to age eighty-one than men who are thirty years old. The statement is true since the eighty-year-old men are no longer at risk of dying between ages thirty and eighty.

There are three major types of comparison errors from which the prospective misrepresenter may choose. Often two or three of them will be used together just to be certain that the reader is impressed by the author's case. This is actually an encouraging thing to know, since the more errors there are, the easier they are to spot. Examining an article full of statistical errors is a bit like evaluating Congress—you may not be able to pick out all the bad ones, but you can be absolutely certain when the whole group isn't doing anything useful or important.

Lack of a control group. Your charming but errant brother, Edgar, who has been ill for quite some time, is told by his doctor that he has only six months to live. His cancer is unquestionably terminal, based on the results of his computerized axial tomography, multiple X-ray studies, physical examination, and numerous laboratory studies. The doctors have handed him a large prescription for morphine and suggested that he begin making final arrangements. Being a plucky chap, Edgar is not the sort to lie down and await the end watching daily installments of "As the World Turns." He begins doing research and discovers that Dr. Wilhelm Masutaki has had great success treating cancer with homogenized eucalyptus leaves. As Dr. Masutaki puts it, "Have you ever seen a koala bear with cancer?" Edgar is impressed by these claims, especially since he has never even seen a sick koala bear. He boards a plane and flies off to Dr. Masutaki's clinic in Sumatra to drink pureed eucalyptus leaves. Six months later he returns hale, hearty, and enthusiastically working for the movement to introduce eucalyptus extract into municipal water supplies. His astounding recovery is enough to convert you as well, so you alter your will, leaving everything to the Masutaki clinic and join in the political fight.

The scenario described is neither ridiculous nor unreal. It happens every day in relation to questions of health and disease, business, politics, and economics. The dramatic is appealing to human beings, and few things are more dramatic than surviving a medical sentence of death. Anecdotes are fun to read, they have human impact, and they deal with human experiences. Unfortunately, when evaluating the potential benefit of a preventive or corrective measure, anecdotes are useless. They confuse, mislead, and fail to explain what happened to all the people who had similar problems, but who are not represented among the anecdotal tales.

Out of every thousand persons who are told that they are dying of cancer, a substantial number, perhaps fifty to seventy-five, will have received a false diagnosis. The diagnosis of disease always has a margin of error. Another ten or twenty of the group will recover spontaneously, for reasons that are completely obscure and which are unrelated to any therapy given. Thus, of the thousand supposedly terminally ill people, nearly a hundred may recover without eating eucalyptus leaves. Out of a thousand such people who go to Sumatra to take the Masutaki cure, these same hundred will provide firm testimonies to the fact that eucalyptus leaves saved their lives. They will believe it. Their drama will be very impressive to themselves, their families, and friends. But unless a new therapy is given in a controlled way to one group and not to another group, *which is otherwise identical to the first group,* it is not possible to determine whether or not the therapy works. Those hundred stories of recovery may make an impressive and convincing book, but without such a comparison or control group, they mean nothing.

Over the years, claims have been made that people with chronic low-back pain are poorly motivated, weak willed, and looking for an easy way out. Similar claims have been made about drug addicts and alcoholics as well as the mentally ill. Controlled studies have subsequently disproved these unfortunate ideas. But when we see an alcoholic who is weak willed we may still have a tendency to blame the alcoholism on this characteristic. Is job motivation different among such persons? Do they suffer from more instability and dissatisfaction in their work? Controlled studies suggest that they may not.

How does one determine if a given program or treatment is successful? Weight loss groups, alcoholic treatment programs, and smoking cessation clinics often make extravagant claims, but unless controlled evaluation is performed, the validity of those claims is subject to doubt. So, when claims for the success of some health regimen are made, ask yourself "Is there a control or comparison group?"

Incorrect control group. Selecting a control group isn't quite enough. As we discussed earlier, we can't reasonably compare death rates from stroke in a community of elderly persons with the same rate in a large city and be able to draw meaningful conclusions about the respective health situations in the two locations. In this instance the problem is that the comparison group is not appropriate. It is too unlike the other group to permit valid interpretation of the results.

A real example of this problem was published several years ago in the *Journal of the American Medical Association.* The study investigated the relationship between heart disease and heredity. It was determined that persons who had heart disease were more likely to have had parents and brothers and sisters who died of heart disease than did the members of a control group who did not have heart disease. The authors concluded that heredity played a large role in determining who got heart disease and who did not. Now, if the control group had been properly selected, this conclusion would at least be potentially correct. However, the authors provided data in their paper indicating that nearly twice as many of the controls had brothers or sisters who died in infancy as did the heart disease cases. Many more of the controls had parents or siblings who had died of accidents and violence. These facts produced two fallacies. First, since the death rate among brothers and sisters of the control group during youth and early adulthood was much higher, these early-death family members did not live long enough to become susceptible to death from heart disease, even though they may have had a predisposition to it. Second, the high death rate among control families for accidents and violence strongly suggests that there was a major difference in socioeconomic status between the cases and the controls. Since we already know that heart disease is related to socioeconomic status, it is possible that the observed differences were due not to heredity, but to those socioeconomic differences.

There are methods by which these deficiencies could have been corrected. For example, the groups could have been subdivided by economic status and each subgroup compared separately. There are also statistical techniques, called adjustments, which can correct for these differences. But in the above example they were not used, and the authors appeared oblivious to the need for them. Therefore, once you have noted that a control group is present, ask yourself, "Is the control group similar to the study group in all important respects?"

Improper generalization. This time you are the minister of health of a small island nation in the central Indian Ocean. Once each month the mail boat brings you your copy of the *American Journal of Public Health,* a magazine which helps you to keep current on major public health issues. This time your journal has been delayed by three days because it had been mistakenly routed to the minister of highways and dams who, having nothing else to do, read it from cover to cover before sending it on. Beside one of the articles he has jotted the words, "Perhaps we should do something about this?"

You begin reading the article. As you proceed, your attention becomes increasingly aroused. A massive and deadly health problem exists which you were unaware of. The article discusses the major health problems in the United States and Canada and points out that there are different ways to view the statistics. In particular, it explains that although heart disease, cancer, and stroke constitute the three leading causes of death, they are not the major cause of years of life lost. Because automobile accidents strike the young more often than the old, a death from an accident in a twenty-five-year-old produces about forty-five lost years of life, whereas a heart disease death at age sixty-eight produces only three or four lost years of life, statistically speaking. If you multiply the average years of life lost times the number of deaths, it turns out that car accidents are the number one killer!

As minister of health you are galvanized to action. Here is the opportunity to wipe out the leading cause of lost years of life using appropriate action. You immediately petition the government to ban private automobiles, build a subway, and subsidize public buses and boats. The prime minister pats you gently on the shoulder and suggests that you cancel your subscription to the *American Journal of Public Health*. You, of course, are outraged at the blind stupidity of politics and government. You resign your post in a flurry of indignation and retire to one of the more remote islands to write your memoirs.

It doesn't require a biostatistician to see that your error as minister of health was to generalize statistics from a highly urbanized society—which uses the automobile as the major means of transport—to your island republic where there are only sixty-two miles of roads and 423 private automobiles. When statistics are gathered, they are usually collected on a small sample of a total population, or, in some instances, on the total population. If they are collected on a sample of the population with the idea of inferring the results to the entire population, the sample must be strictly representative of the total group, as has already been discussed. No matter how well the sample of auto accident deaths represented the United States and Canada, it was not representative of the population of your island. Thus, statistical inferences are possible only when the group for which you are generalizing the result resembles the group that was studied.

Further, statistics referring to the "average" do not apply to persons who clearly differ from that average by a substantial degree, and the addition of more information may make a reasonable inference invalid. For example, studies indicate that the average forty-five-year-old man has a 7.5 percent chance of developing heart disease over the next eight years. Few of us, however, are average. If you go to a doctor and have your cholesterol and blood sugar levels tested, take an electrocardiogram, and tell him how many cigarettes you smoke each day, he can put that information together into a personal estimate of risk. Using that information alone (and certainly other factors could be considered), your risk of heart disease over the next eight years after age forty-five can vary from 2.2 percent to 77.8 percent.[1] Both of these figures assume that no heart disease exists at the time of the examination.

Population-based statistics often have little personal validity unless they are greatly subdivided into categories that closely resemble your circumstances. Knowing that cigarettes can cause lung cancer, for example, is enormously helpful to persons trying to formulate policies designed to reduce the incidence of cancer in the population, but the fact that cigarette smokers have approximately ten times as much lung cancer as nonsmokers says very little about you personally. If you smoke a lot, the risk is greater; if you smoke less, risk is correspondingly less. Beware of generalizing averages to your own case. Always ask yourself, "Are the results generalized to groups similar enough to the study group to justify the generalization?"

3. Using the wrong statistics. You have reached the pinnacle of success in the health world. Your position, while lofty, is often an ephemeral one. You like being Secretary of Health and Human Services, though, and are accordingly anxious to solve all major health crises quickly. One of your aides sends a report indicating that in 1920 the proportionate mortality (the percent of all deaths due to a given cause) for congenital malformations was 6 percent for persons dying before one year of age. That is, of all babies that died, 6 percent died of congenital malformation. In 1960, the proportionate mortality due to congenital malformations was 14 percent. Your aide has submitted a brief with these statistics, pointing out that several experts have attributed this increase in death from congenital malformations to such things as radioactive fallout, LSD, X-rays, and pesticides. He urges a massive campaign to decrease our exposure to these toxic environmental hazards.

As secretary you find the statistics quite compelling and disturbing, but you are uneasy at using them to reorganize your health priorities. The fallout issue is especially sensitive, since the administration is straining to remain neutral in the nuclear energy battle. The pesticide problem is equally difficult. Neutrality is the key to political survival, and your aide is definitely pushing you out on a limb. You decide to get some advice and phone the department of epidemiology at Johns Hopkins School of Public Health. A second-year student answers the office phone, explaining that everyone has already gone home for the evening. In desperation you describe your problem to her.

"So?" she replies with a tone of maddening superiority. (Epidemiologists learn to talk with maddening superiority at an early stage in their training.) "What are the infant death rates for 1920 and 1960?"

"I just gave them to you," you mutter impatiently.

"No, you didn't," she says. "You gave me the proportionate mortality rates, the percent of all deaths due to a given cause. The death rate is the total number of deaths divided by the population."

You grab a volume from the National Center for Health Statistics and search out the requested information.

"In 1920 the death rate under one year of age was 85.8 per thousand persons. In 1960 it was 26.0 per thousand."

"I thought so," she says. "Give me just a minute while I do some figuring."

Hurriedly she constructs table 6.2. After a few moments she chuckles and suggests that maybe she ought to be Health and Human Services Secretary.

TABLE 6.2
Use of Proportionate Mortality and Overall Death Rate to Calculate Death Rate Increase Due to Congenital Malformations

	Proportionate mortality due to congenital malformations	Infant death rate	Death rate from congenital malformations
1920	6%	85.8 per 1,000	5.1 per 1,000
1960	14%	26.0 per 1,000	3.6 per 1,000

"You see," she crows, "in 1920, 6 percent of those 85.8 deaths were due to congenital malformations. That is, about 5.1 babies under one year of age died for every thousand births. In 1960, 14 percent of the 26.0 deaths, or 3.6 per thousand babies, died from congenital malformations. Thus the death rate or risk of dying from congenital malformation was only about two-thirds as great in 1960 as it was in 1920. The higher proportional mortality is due to the fact that other causes of death have decreased even more, leaving congenital malformations with a slightly larger fraction of a smaller total. You used the wrong statistic to draw your conclusion."

This example is taken from real data. The conclusions about radioactive fallout and pesticides are similar to conclusions reached every day by authors and readers who select the wrong statistic to prove a point. This is an extremely common trap and one which will often fool even a sophisticated reader who is not alert to the problem.

Another example, taken from the journal *California Medicine*, concerns a report on four hundred suicides in San Mateo County during the years 1961 to 1965. The authors noted that widows constituted 15 percent of the suicides and widowers only 5 percent "suggesting that males better tolerate the loss of their marital partners." Table 6.3 provides census data for San Mateo County not included in the article. It obviously never

TABLE 6.3
San Mateo County (California) 1960 Census Data

	Male	Female
Single	30,735	24,778
Married	111,948	112,101
Widowed	3,227	15,116
Divorced	4,161	7,053
	150,071	158,548

occurred to the authors that there might have been more suicides among widows because there were more widows. In fact, while three times as many suicides occur among widows, there are nearly five times as many widows as widowers. What is required here is the suicide *rate* among widows and widowers, not the proportion of suicides in each group. The suicide rate among widows is equal to $400 \times .15/15,116 = .004$ (or 4 per thousand widows). The comparable rate among widowers is $400 \times .05/3,227 = .006$ (or 6 per thousand widowers). Thus, a widower is one and one-half times more likely to commit suicide in San Mateo County than is a widow, the opposite of the authors' conclusion.

Always ask yourself, "Are these the appropriate statistics for arriving at the conclusion given?"

4. Asking the unanswerable questions. Suppose you find in your mailbox a survey questionnaire from something billed as the National Study on Health Promotion (NSHP). You are asked to complete the questionnaire in the interests of further-ing medical science's understanding of the factors which cause disease. Being a good citizen, you decide to comply. Included among the long array of items are these three questions: (1) In what state or country were you born? (2) How old are you? and (3) If married, how often have you had extramarital sexual re-lationships? Obviously, these questions range from a relatively neutral item about birthplace to the highly sensitive area of illi-cit sexual behavior. Will these three questions be answered with equal reliability? Probably not.

The National Health Survey, a periodic federal survey of the state of health of the American people, was interested in deter-mining how valid the answers to its questions were. During 1954–55 they selected a large sample of persons in Baltimore to complete the health interview. The interviewers were skilled and spent a good deal of time with each individual. In the course of the interview they inquired about each person's medi-cal history. Later, the members of the sample received a diag-nostic medical evaluation and the results of the home interview were compared to those from the medical evaluation. Table 6.4 indicates the frequency of the reporting of various medical con-ditions on the interview compared to the physical examination findings.

Some conditions were much better reported than others. Asthma, hay fever, chronic sinus problems, and chronic bron-chitis were reported more often by interview than by physical examination. The other conditions examined were greatly underreported. The critical point in this example is that the

TABLE 6.4
Frequency of Various Illnesses as Reported in the
National Health Survey Interview of 1954–55 and as
Determined by Medical Evaluation of the Same Individuals

Selected chronic conditions	Household interview	Evaluation diagnosis
(1)	(2)	(3)
	Rate per 1,000 population	Rate per 1,000 population
Heart conditions	21.8	91.7
High blood pressure	32.9	66.4
Diabetes	10.7	26.9
Peptic ulcer	2.4	8.7
Arthritis and rheumatism	43.7	79.9
Hernia	8.5	38.8
Asthma–hay fever	38.9	30.0
Chronic bronchitis	14.6	10.1
Chronic sinusitis	21.7	12.8

person asked the question may not know the true answer. He or she may be unaware of early diabetes, a heart murmur, or a hernia. However, if the question is sensitive, for example, if it deals with mental illness or sexual practices, the interviewee may know the answer but be unwilling to divulge it.

Finally, the means used to identify positive or negative responses is critical. Table 6.5 shows the reported rates of diabetes

TABLE 6.5
Diabetes Prevalence in Studies with Physical Examinations
Compared to United States Estimate (Rates per 1,000 population)

Area of survey of estimate	Year	Crude rate	Adjusted rate*
Oxford, Mass.	1946–1947	17.5	21.2
New Market, Ont.	1949	12.2	18.8
Baltimore, Md.	1953–1955	16.7	23.0
United States prevalence estimate	1958		16.9

*Adjusted according to the distribution of the 1957 population of U.S. by race and broad age groups.

in three United States cities and in the entire nation for different years. The highest figure exceeds the lowest by 36 percent. Are the differences real? To answer that question, one must know how diabetes was defined in the different studies. Was it determined by the presence of diabetic symptoms or by the level of blood sugar in a fasting individual, or was it based on the more detailed and expensive glucose tolerance test? If based on laboratory studies, what values were used as cut-off points for determining whether or not a given individual had diabetes? Were these cut-off points the same in each study?

In this example, differences in definition of diabetes were great enough that the results of the studies cannot be meaningfully compared. Each may be accurate, each may include completely precise and usable information, but the definitions differ. The comparisons are invalid.

Always ask "Can the information presented really be accurately obtained?" and "Were the same criteria applied to all comparison groups?"

5. Misinterpretation. You are a plastic surgeon specializing in the treatment and repair of cleft palate, and you decide to see if you can determine if there are any maternal characteristics that seem to be associated with the birth of a child having a cleft palate. You have read an article about common errors in designing a study and decide that the data you collect will be highly accurate. You establish rigorous and reproducible criteria for identifying cleft palate and design a brief questionnaire to be given to mothers of children with cleft palates. Table 6.6 presents your results (the data are real, taken from the medical journal *Plastic and Reconstructive Surgery*). You conclude (the conclusions also taken from the same journal) that "the high incidence of cleft palate in the first born may be attributed to the severe anxiety frequently associated with the first pregnancy, coupled with other stressful situations."

Conclusions such as this are a good source of banner headlines in the tabloid press. To the uncritical they are persuasive,

TABLE 6.6
Cleft Palate in 228 Children

Incident of Cleft Palate	Number of Children	Percent
Incidence of cleft palate in first-born	92	40
Incidence of cleft palate in second-born	62	27
Incidence of cleft palate in third-born	43	19
Incidence of cleft palate in fourth to sixteenth-born	31	14
		100

but if you have been following this chapter closely you should detect several error types. First, the conclusion attributing cleft palate to the anxiety of first pregnancy is not based on any of the data presented. This is a common ploy of propagandists and politicians. "The crime rate is rising. Elect me and it will go down." Similar statements are often juxtaposed, and we seldom stop to ask ourselves how the proposed solution relates to what may be a real problem. Second, association and cause are not equivalent. There are more ice cream bars sold at the beach on days when there are more drownings. The association is strong, but few people would blame the drownings on the ice cream. Nevertheless, we often set policy in just such a way.

In addition to this conclusion based on insufficient information (error type 1), a comparison error is also present. First-born children with cleft palate have been compared to second-born children with cleft palate, when they ought to be compared to first-born children without cleft palate if factors associated with the occurrence of cleft palate are sought (error type 2).

Third, although the table indicates that the incidence of cleft palate has been calculated by birth order, the addition of these percentages (not shown in the original journal article) totals 100 percent, making it clear that this figure is not incidence at all, but rather the percent of all children with cleft palate who were first-born, second-born, and so on. Incidence by contrast is strictly defined as follows:

$$\text{Incidence} = \frac{\text{Number of new cases of a disease over a given time}}{\text{Total population}}$$

Incidence is *not* the same as prevalence, although it is frequently misused that way:

$$\text{Prevalence} = \frac{\text{Number of existing cases now}}{\text{Total population}}$$

Incidence is, in fact, the statistic needed to measure risk of cleft palate by birth order. But it has not been calculated in this study. To do so, it is necessary to calculate the number of cases over a given time (say a year) of cleft palate in first-born children divided by the number of first-born children. About 40 percent of all births are first births. Therefore, it is not surprising that 40 percent of cleft palates occur among the first born. Cleft palates have no relation to birth order and, when properly examined, these data reveal that fact. Thus, there is an error of type 3 (using the wrong statistics) as well.

It is neither necessary nor desirable for nonresearchers to become experts in the methodology of study design and interpretation. It is, however, useful to keep these five error types in mind. Refer again to Table 6.1; keep it handy for reference the next time you read about something that is supposed to be good for you or not good for you. It is reasonable to take action to protect yourself from only those things which appear dangerous after rigorous testing has produced relatively consistent findings.

We know enough to say with reasonable certainty that we ought to eat a diet lower in fat, to be slim, to exercise regularly, to control high blood pressure, to avoid cigarettes, and to get a reasonable amount of fiber in our diet. We should eat less sugar and wear seat belts when we drive. Undoubtedly, there are many other things we can do to improve our health, but the suggestions listed here are sound, safe, and supported by lots of test information.

Chapter 7
Screening for Disease

Do You Really Need
That Annual Pap Smear?

I say one thing, you write another, and those who read you understand still something else.

—*Nikos Kazantzakis*

Ask a physician how he or she helps prevent disease and chances are that the reply will center around annual physical examinations, Pap smears for women, and assorted laboratory tests designed to detect the presence of illness at an early stage. Immunization may be mentioned as well. Vaccines represent genuine efforts to prevent disease, but disease screening is not a preventive measure at all. It is aimed at early detection of illness under the notion that most illness can be more successfully treated when identified early.

This distinction, which may seem picky at first glance, is really quite fundamental. Early detection does not address cause at all. If it increases the likelihood of cure (which it may or may not), it still bears no relation to the probability that a similar illness will strike again. This chapter, then, is not about prevention. It concerns the time and costs, both economic and psychologic, of detecting disease at an early stage.

A screening test is simply a means of dividing people into two groups: those who may have a given disease and those who do not have that disease. It is *not* meant to be a definitive diagnosis, but rather to limit the number of persons who should receive more thorough diagnostic testing. Misunderstanding of this fact has led to a great deal of misery and psychological trauma—which ought to be reckoned in estimating the costs of such procedures. Most of the people who have a positive serologic test for syphilis, for example, do not have syphilis. Explaining that to the satisfaction of an irate spouse, however, can be difficult and challenging.

The problem is that not everything can be fitted into "either/ or" categories. Ideally, screening tests would divide the sick and the well as they do in figure 7.1. All the diseased persons fall to the right of the dashed vertical line, all the well people to the left of it. In reality, no screening tests give results that are so

FIGURE 7.1
Performance of a "Perfect" Screening Test

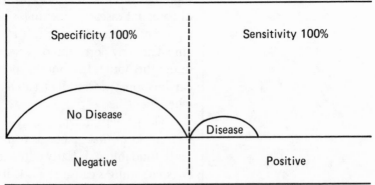

SOURCE: Adapted from M. Henderson, "Validity of Screening," *Cancer* 37 (1976): 573-81. Reprinted with permission of the author and publisher.

clear-cut. Figure 7.2 is a far more realistic example of how screening tests behave. There is an overlap of test results of the well and the sick, represented by the area between the two vertical dashed lines. If the screening test is to the left of (lower than) vertical line 1, no disease is present. If it is to the right of line 2, disease is clearly present. But one-fourth of healthy people and one-half of sick people in this example score between the lines. The relative numbers of sick and well within this range will also depend on how common the disease is. In general, those who are well vastly outnumber those who are not. Therefore, most persons who have a positive screening test for a disease do *not* actually have the disease.

Three measures are used to determine the efficacy of a screening test in detecting disease:

1. Sensitivity. Sensitivity is the fraction of all persons who have a given disease who also have a positive screening test. If

FIGURE 7.2
Performance of a Realistic Screening Test

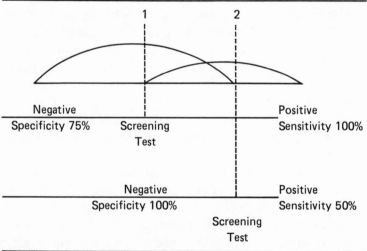

SOURCE: Adapted from M. Henderson, "Validity of Screening," *Cancer* 37 (1976): 573–81. Reprinted with permission of the author and publisher.

100 persons with a given condition are tested and 70 have positive screening tests, then the sensitivity of that test is 70 percent.

2. Specificity. The specificity of a test is the fraction of all persons without a given condition (i.e., healthy people) who have a negative screening test. If 100 healthy persons receive a test and 90 of them have negative tests, then the specificity is 90 percent.

3. Predictive value. The predictive value of a test is the fraction of all positive tests for a condition which actually represents true disease. If 100 persons have positive tests, but only 50 of them actually have disease, then the predictive value of the test is 50 percent. The predictive value of a test depends on sensitivity, specificity, and prevalence of the disease in question. Unfortunately, this measure of the efficacy of a screening test is often neglected, although it is the single most critical means for determining the usefulness of a screening test in identifying a disease. Very rare diseases will have low predictive values even if they have a high specificity and sensitivity. For example, suppose a screening test has a sensitivity of 100 percent (100 percent of all persons with disease have positive tests), a specificity of 95 percent (95 percent of persons without disease have a negative test), and a prevalence in the population of one new case for every 10,000 tests. Let us further suppose that the disease is 100 percent fatal unless it is identified at an early stage. The test costs only $3 and the treatment, when disease is found, costs only $300. The only harmful effect of the treatment is that 1 in 500 persons treated dies from an allergic reaction.

Since this test is superior to many which are currently available, it is likely that it would be in general use. However, consider the following: of every 10,000 persons tested (on the average), one actual case will be identified. 500 false positives will also be identified and treated, and one of these people will die. The total monetary costs will be $10.000 \times 3 = \$30,000$ for screening, and $501 \times 300 = \$150,300$ for treatment. One life will have been saved and one life lost. The low prevalence of the disease means that the vast majority of positive tests will occur in well persons. The predictive value of the test will be approximately 1/500 or 0.2 percent.

The World Health Organization has outlined criteria which screening tests ought to meet before they are used.[1] They are:

1. The condition sought is an important health problem.
2. There is an accepted treatment for patients with recognized disease.
3. Facilities for diagnosis and treatment are available.
4. There is a recognizable latent or early symptomatic stage.
5. There is a suitable test or examination.
6. The test is acceptable to the population.
7. The natural history of the condition, including development from latent to declared disease, is adequately understood.
8. There is an agreed policy about whom to treat as patients.
9. The cost of case finding (including diagnosis and treatment of patients diagnosed) is economically balanced in relation to possible expenditure on medical care as a whole.
10. Case-finding is a continuing process and not a "once and for all" project.

Ironically, the authors concluded that none of the common screening tests in use during the 1960s, when the criteria were developed, met all of the above conditions. The *Lancet*, a British medical journal, carried a long series of articles during 1974 which reviewed screening procedures then available. They concluded that a few were probably useful, but the majority of routine screening tests were probably not very beneficial.

All of this confusion does not exist because researchers or doctors have been irresponsible or because there is some kind of sinister plot to foist bad medical care on the population and use unneeded medical services to enrich the coffers of wealthy corporations. Statistics are often used to lie to us; at other times they seem contradictory, even if presented with the greatest sincerity. But for certain kinds of decisions, statistics are the only means for drawing reasonable conclusions. Countless times I have heard physicians reject sound evidence because something else once worked for them. The personal is more meaningful than the statistical in shaping our decisions. At times this is appropriate. But when we are attempting to select an approach to a problem which has the highest probability of success, statistics, which are based on estimates of probability, are the soundest method of decision-making.

In the real world, though, there are many uncertainties. Studies may be done to evaluate a screening test, for example, and the results may be inconclusive. Public policy of all sorts must often be made against a background of uncertainty.

THE PAP SMEAR

Perhaps the commonest screening test used today is the Pap smear, otherwise known as cervical cytology. Soon after entering adolescence most women begin having Pap smears on a regular basis for the remainder of their lives. These tests are designed to identify cancer of the cervix, one of the most common forms of cancer in women. The test allows the detection of early malignant and even "premalignant" changes in the cervix at a stage when cure is essentially certain. Since the early 1950s when the Pap smear became widely used death rates from cervical cancer have declined steadily, and this has been used as a strong argument in support of the efficacy of the Pap smear. Earlier, I noted a decline in the cancer death rate prior to 1950, many years *before* the introduction of the Pap smear. Does this mean that the smear is ineffective? Not at all, but it certainly gives rise to some questions.

One of the questions that gradually has been answered deals with the discrepancy between the relatively large numbers of "premalignant" findings on the Pap test and the much smaller numbers of cancers that eventually become symptomatic. An argument has raged over whether these findings are of genuinely premalignant cells, or if they simply represent transient inflammation. It is now generally believed that premalignancies are reversible, but that they occasionally proceed to malignancy. It is clear that, if they do become malignant, there is a long period of latency. The annual Pap smear, a part of American medical dogma for thirty years, no longer needs to be annual, according to recent recommendations of the National Cancer Institute and the American Cancer Society.[2]

The Pap test is still recommended, but for low-risk women (no prior history of disease, normal previous Pap tests, no symptoms), it need not be done more than once every two or three years. And its efficacy is still uncertain. The literature on Pap tests is filled with studies that appear to contradict each other. This reflects the general problem of trying to evaluate something that has an expected benefit only in the very long term and in only a relatively few of those who go through the procedure.

DECISION-MAKING IN THE FACE OF UNCERTAINTY

There are times when we must make decisions in the face of uncertainty. No matter how much we might like definitive answers, they simply aren't available. In their absence we can: (1) write the choices down on a piece of paper, hang the paper on the wall, throw a dart at it, and select the option struck by the dart; (2) take the choice that "sounds" best; (3) ask a friend which to choose; or (4) examine the data and pick the one that looks best on the basis of available information. In real life, few follow the last course of action. Las Vegas and Atlantic City survive and profit by assuming that people will not play the odds. If you play the odds, you are banned from their casinos.

Because if you are careful in your choices, you will always win in the long run, despite losing now and then as you go along.

E. George Knox spoke of the uncertainties surrounding Pap smears to a conference of cytologists in Italy:

> If there were no uncertainties concerning the essential elements of the theoretical background it would in principle be possible to calculate the consequences of any given planning proposal. That is, given that the frequency and ages of the screening procedure were declared, the outcome in terms of cases proceeding to invasion and numbers of women dying, should be calculable. Furthermore, it should be possible to compare the results of alternative policies, including a policy of no screening at all and thus, at each stage of a growing service, to calculate the extra benefit to be obtained from each extra investment. If the calculations were easy it would be possible to examine every possible policy against every possible set of alternative premises and so cover the ranges of uncertainty within which each policy would need to be assessed.[3]

Because uncertainties exist, policy must be created by selecting the choice which available information suggests has the greatest probability of success. Current recommendations with respect to Pap smears represent such a best choice. Few screening tests, however, have been scrutinized as thoroughly as the Pap smear.

TYPES OF SCREENING PROCEDURES

Many different approaches to the detection of early disease have been used. Up to this point I have been discussing individual procedures designed to detect specific conditions at an early stage. At least two other approaches are in widespread use: multiphasic screening and health hazard appraisal.

Multiphasic screening is an outgrowth of the acceptance by

many health practitioners of the value of screening in general, and the notion that there can't be too much of a good thing. It also provides a means for doing a relatively thorough health inventory without expensive physician services. The annual physical examination is time consuming, expensive, wasteful of both physician and patient time, and its efficacy in reducing illness is largely unproven. Multiphasic screening is designed to overcome all of these problems. Instead of one doctor examining one patient, the multiphasic examination usually involves a battery of standard laboratory procedures which are often performed by an inexpensive automated analyzer that can provide dozens of test results from the same small sample of blood. These laboratory studies are often combined with an electrocardiogram, brief examinations of heart, lungs, eyes, and other organ systems by nonphysician technicians, and a printed summary of results. Results are given to patients and, where warranted, pertinent clinical findings are discussed and recommendations made. All this sounds elaborate, highly technological, and impressive.

Only one formal trial of the benefits of this approach has been conducted.[4] This trial involved long-term follow-up of several thousand persons who were given annual multiphasic examinations and a control group that was not urged to have such tests. The results were expectedly vague. A significant reduction of illness and disability was observed only for the oldest age group of men examined (forty-five to fifty-four years of age). The investigators enthusiastically estimated that the lower disability and absentee rates among examined men in that age group amounted to a savings of more than $800 (1972 dollars) a year per man. Another observer commented on the same results this way:

> After several years of the program these investigations were unable to determine any favorable health effect of periodic examinations on women, and only one group of men, between the

ages of forty-five and fifty-four, showed differences in disability and absenteeism. Furthermore, these differences, while statistically significant, are clinically unimpressive—only 3.9 percent less disability and 1.3 percent better attendance at work. The results of this study are quite sobering.[5]

So, you are tempted to ask, what can I make of all this? How can I make sense of multiphasic screening (or anything else) if the investigators, with all their training and research money, cannot do so? Stand back from these results. Researchers often get so enmeshed in the issue of whether or not the differences between two groups are statistically significant that they lose perspective. Multiphasic checkups may, indeed, be beneficial. Perhaps if the scientists had begun with older individuals they might have found even greater significance in their results. One thing is clear, though. These examinations did not result in overwhelming, large-scale alterations in the health and well-being of those studied. The impact of smoking cessation on health compared to these examinations is like comparing a redwood to a cattail. If you smoke two packs a day and arrive faithfully for your annual multiphasic examination, you are deluding yourself into thinking you are taking care of your health. You are not. If you are obese, hypertensive, sedentary, nourished by junk foods high in fats and sugars, no amount of annual testing can remotely compensate for what you are doing to yourself. Save your money.

Health hazard appraisal is a technique developed by two physicians, Jack Hall and Lewis Robbins, of the Methodist Hospital of Indiana. It is an attempt to combine the results of laboratory testing with risk information based on behaviors of various sorts to estimate the specific risk of dying for each person. This technique can be used to give you a physiologic age, as opposed to your calendar age. Thus, if you are thirty-five years old, smoke, have high blood pressure, never use seat belts, and are twenty pounds overweight, you might be told that you are really forty-four in terms of your life expectancy.

There are many problems associated with this technique, but at least it uses information that can be applied preventively to forego the onset of disease. The accuracy of the statistical information has been questioned, as have the approaches used by the plethora of corporations which have appeared on the scene marketing slick risk-information packages to the public. No evidence has been gathered to demonstrate that this approach leads to improvements in health. But if you are the sort of person who might change your ways if it were determined that your body is eight or ten years older than you thought, you might consider getting such an appraisal.

I recently published a review of methods of risk assessment and screening. The conclusion of that review is worth repeating here:

> The value of such activities in promoting health undoubtedly varies and is strongly related both to the characteristics measured and the effort given to implementing needed changes and therapies. Risk assessment without follow-up is of little value; it is also true that changing health-related behaviors, both those of the general public and those of medical practitioners, is a complex and difficult problem that mere concern alone will not solve.[6]

Chapter 8
Evaluating Medical Practice

Did the Shaman Know Something We Don't Know?

Show a man too many camels' bones, or show them to him too often, and he will not be able to recognize a live camel when he sees one.

—*Mirza Ahsan of Tabriz*

In 1860 Georg Ebers discovered an Egyptian papyrus document, dating from the fifteenth century B.C. which revealed that the practice of medicine was astonishingly sophisticated among ancient Egyptians. It is reasonable to assume that the papyrus was based on a centuries-long tradition of medical care and practice. Medicine has long been a central focus of human attention, both because of the suffering which often accompanies illness and because of the almost universal desire to extend life beyond its normal span.

ROOTS OF MEDICAL PRACTICE

The numbers of current medical and particularly pharmaceutical practices with roots extending into the dim past are not insignificant. Aspirin, or acetyl salicylic acid, is one of our commonest drugs. Its botanical parent, salicylic acid, was well known to Hippocrates and was derived from willow bark. Somehow, knowledge of the pain-relieving qualities of willow bark was lost to much of the Western world for nearly fifteen hundred years, only to be rediscovered in the sixteenth or seventeenth century by practicing physicians. (There is some evidence that practicing homemakers, however, never stopped brewing their willow bark teas.)

Surgery to remove painful bladder stones has been practiced, if rather mercilessly, for thousands of years. Digitalis preparations derived from the foxglove plant—as they have been for centuries—are still used to sustain lives of persons with failing hearts. Quinine is still an effective, if no longer optimal, treatment for malaria, and this wonder drug was prepared from cinchona bark by South American Indians long before the Spanish Conquest.

The catalog of modern medical applications of ancient medical knowledge has filled books. Nevertheless, few physicians get through medical school without hearing the common estimate that it was not until the second decade of the twentieth century that a patient had more chance of being helped by a physician than harmed. If this is true, how could the profession have flourished so remarkably through all those thousands of years? Is it possible that those ancient wise men, so often quoted, harmed more than they helped? Was Hippocrates a hypocrite? Was the Roman genius, Galen, whose views dominated medicine for more than a thousand years after his death, a fraud?

It is probably not possible to answer such questions directly. Certainly, such men did contribute significantly to our understanding of how the human body works. Hippocrates was acutely mindful that the primary charge to a physician was "first, do no harm."

From early times Western physicians were viewed as healers. In contrast physicians of the Far East were seen as maintainers of health and received payment from patients only so long as they remained well. The Western attitude focused medical attention on disease, rather than health, from an early time. The scientific revolution of the eighteenth and nineteenth centuries led to the experimental search for new approaches to healing, which directly produced the vast changes in medical care that have characterized this century. Since this revolution was primarily laboratory based, the advances in theory and technique were seldom systematically tested once they were applied to human populations. The epidemiologic approach to studying cause was applied to public health, but the methods of research design developed to understand large-scale effects of various therapies were only infrequently applied to newly emerging technologies and therapeutic practices. Instead, announcements of new medical treatments were usually greeted with wild enthusiasm and adopted on a large scale, rapidly becoming the community standards of practice. If the therapeutic practice had serious enough side effects or was ineffective in most persons, disillusionment set in. Eventually, a standard set of indications for a therapy would be adopted, and it would achieve a stable place in the physician's armamentarium.

THE ROLE OF
MEDICAL SCHOOLS

Attending a medical school can be little different from studying at a school of theology. One is usually taught that "this is the way things are." Deviations from the norm are not tolerated. Strangely enough, despite the very real problems physicians have with unwarranted medical malpractice cases in the United States, I have heard more frequent and assured insinuations of malpractice from physicians than from any other group. Several years ago, I headed a group that wrote a grant proposal to study the potential uses of relaxation and meditation in lowering risk factors for heart disease. In the course of events, the proposal was reviewed by the committee for the protection of human subjects at the hospital in San Francisco where I was working at the time. The study involved persons with marginally elevated blood pressures and it contained an escape clause stating that persons with a diastolic blood pressure (pressure when the heart is in its relaxation phase) of 95 mm Hg (mercury) or greater at two successive visits would be placed on conventional medical therapy. One of the physicians on the committee disapproved the study because "it is malpractice to medically treat any person with a diastolic blood pressure below 100 mm Hg." Another of the committee members disapproved the study because "it is medical malpractice not to treat any person with a diastolic blood pressure above 90 mm Hg." Both physicians accused the protocol of departing from conventional standards of medical therapy in the community, and yet their statements were diametrically opposed. They did not discuss or even seem concerned about this discrepancy, but merely agreed that the study should be disapproved because it was unsafe.

This dogmatic interpretation, that "malpractice is anything I don't do," has led to a rigidity in medical care that has prevented adequate evaluation of most therapeutic practices. The beginnings of this dogmatism lie in the almost exclusive acceptance of compulsive grade seekers into medical schools. But it is nurtured into full blossom in the sterile academic environments which characterize most teaching medical centers. The extreme emphasis on technical skill to the exclusion of interpersonal relationships has succeeded in greatly reducing the efficacy of the most effective tool ancient medicine had, the placebo effect.

THE PLACEBO EFFECT

Placebos are inactive drugs or therapies often given in place of active treatment to control groups in studies that define the effectiveness of a new therapy. It is necessary to give such placebos because of the fact that merely receiving some form of therapy, regardless of its known effectiveness, results in improvement for some people. Often, this effect is mistakenly labeled "imaginary" or "all in the mind," with the derisive implication that the individual who has benefited from the placebo was making up the symptoms in the first place.

This implication is false. Shamans and witch doctors for thousands of years have known that doing something, anything, is better than doing nothing. Doctors know it, too. They prescribe antibiotics for viral colds when they know full well that the medication won't kill the germ causing the cold. They prescribe drugs for pain which in clinical testing perform no better than placebos in relieving pain. Frequently, patients will say that only this particular drug relieves the pain. Despite the drug's high cost, the physician may well prescribe it knowing that it is working as a placebo. Is the patient better off having an effective placebo (if it is safe) than being disabused of the notion that the drug is effective and being left with nothing to believe in? Placebo effects are real. One can measure changes in blood pressure, gastric acid secretion, heart rate, and other physiological processes after the administration of placebos. They work, and because they work, it is not possible to determine the effectiveness of an active therapy without comparison to a placebo.

Needless to say, this raises ethical questions which many physicians would like to avoid. The simplest way to avoid these questions, then, is to simply accept without testing. Avoiding these questions has led to the problems discussed below. Surely countless others, as yet unevaluated, await future discovery.

THERAPEUTIC ERRORS
IN MODERN MEDICINE

Internal Mammary Artery Ligation

Angina pectoris is a condition resulting from an inadequate blood supply to the heart muscle. In persons who have severe atherosclerosis (hardening of the arteries) in the arteries supplying the heart, fatty, calcified debris called plaque may gradually occlude these vessels. Because the artery becomes progressively smaller in diameter, the affected individual may experience pain with exercise. This pain results from the fact that exercise increases the need for oxygen to meet the additional demand on the heart. A person with angina cannot get sufficient blood through the narrowed vessels to meet these increased demands, and chest pain results. A brief rest leads to the subsidence of pain, but renewed activity brings it back. As time proceeds, the level of activity needed to cause pain may become less and less until almost total disability occurs.

It had long been known that several arteries in the chest give rise to small collateral vessels which communicate with the coronary arteries and that these connections will enlarge if the main artery from which they branch is tied off, or ligated. In 1939 an Italian physician extended this knowledge by reasoning that ligating the internal mammary artery should result in improved blood flow to the heart through these enlarging collateral vessels. He performed the surgery on a patient who did well and experienced relief of pain and who was reported well two years after the procedure. Still, it wasn't until 1955 that a large series of cases were reported. Of seventy-five cases, sixty-four were reported alive and improved after internal mammary artery ligation. A group of Philadelphia surgeons picked up on this remarkable success and, within eighteen months, had completed an additional one hundred fifty surgeries using the same technique. About two-thirds of these were pain-free or significantly improved in the months following surgery. Other investigators rapidly added additional cases, the results seeming to be consistent everywhere: high rate of improvement, low fatality rates, and even improved electrocardiograms.

Still, a few surgeons were concerned by the fact that dog studies could not demonstrate significantly improved coronary circulation after ligation of the internal mammary arteries and also that no controlled trials had ever been done.

In the face of the overwhelming tide toward adopting the procedure, a small group of investigators decided to do a placebo controlled trial. In this instance, "placebo" meant sham operation; half the patients had the internal mammary arteries exposed and ligated and half had them exposed but not ligated. Now, there are ethical questions surrounding this study. People were exposed to the risks of surgery and to its attendant discomfort and anxiety without receiving any active therapy. It is doubtful that the study could be performed at the present time. But the results were rather startling. The actively treated group and the placebo group did equally well. A few persons in each group had electrocardiographic changes after the surgery, confirming that real physiologic change can result from a placebo procedure and also confirming that angina pectoris has an especially great potential for responding to placebo treatments. Unlike the other trials, these patients were followed for long periods of time. In neither group did the beneficial results last for more than a few months. Thus, internal mammary artery ligation died an early death and, because of a questionably ethical study, tens of thousands of persons over the following years were saved the risks, discomfort, and cost of this procedure.

Amphetamines and Weight Loss

Each of us has a list of things we would like to do but are not doing. For millions of Americans weight loss is at the top of that list. The determinants of human behaviors are many and varied, and changing our daily routines is extraordinarily difficult. Most smokers want to quit smoking, but they don't. Most people who are overweight would like to lose that extra weight, but they don't. "If only there were a pill," they often say to themselves. For the weight conscious there are pills. The only trouble is that they don't work. The drug companies who make so much money selling these pills forget to emphasize what happens to people who take amphetamines and their newer, somewhat safer cousins. It took controlled trials comparing weight loss from amphetamines to that from placebos and also to the effects of diet alone to detect the true effects.

Amphetamines work by suppressing appetite. This they do effectively—at least for a short time. A person who begins taking diet pills will eat less for a couple of weeks and notice some weight loss. This, plus the fact that these pills, in the words of George Carlin, "make you grind your teeth and feel good," tends to reinforce their continued use. In the long run, however, persons taking these pills gain weight rather than lose it, and they certainly do worse than persons using diet alone to control their weight problem. They also have pronounced and frequently negative side effects which can creep up on the user. Easy answers have a propensity for being inadequate answers.

Enteric-Coated Potassium

High blood pressure, or hypertension, is one of the commonest medical conditions of middle age. It is associated with significant elevations in risk of heart attack, stroke, and kidney disease. The first line of medical therapy for hypertension usually involves a class of drugs called diuretics. These drugs reduce blood pressure by increasing the amount of fluid which is excreted by the kidneys. Letting extra fluid escape from the vascular system reduces pressure in the same way that letting air out of a tire lowers the pressure in the tire.

A side effect of these drugs involves an excess loss of the

necessary chemical potassium along with the fluid loss. Often, persons who take diuretics must take additional potassium in order to make up for this loss. As medicine, potassium leaves something to be desired. It tastes terrible and must be taken on a regular basis. Because of this, many persons who are supposed to take it in the form of a liquid frequently skip doses. To increase the palatability of potassium, a form of the drug called enteric-coated potassium was developed. This was designed to work like the "tiny time pills" advertised in cold-remedy commercials. The drug is concentrated and surrounded by a slowly dissolving cover designed to gradually release the potassium into the intestinal tract. The idea seemed a good one, the medication was a safe one, and the pills were produced for the market in the early 1960s with little clinical testing.

Slowly, reports began to accumulate of persons with recurrent abdominal pain, associated with weight loss and vomiting. The pains tended to increase over a period of months, often leading to intestinal obstruction and even perforation of the intestinal wall. Surgical intervention identified ulcers and scars on the intestinal wall farther down than they usually occur. A review of cases eventually identified the fact that all of the involved persons had hypertension, were taking diuretics, and had enteric-coated potassium supplements to replace lost potassium supplies. A survey of 440 hospitals eventually revealed 275 cases and 15 deaths associated with these enteric-coated tablets. It seemed these early pills released their potassium much too rapidly, leading to irritation and ulceration of the intestinal lining.

Although the cause of the problem was clearly identified as a nonessential toxic drug, the drug was not removed from the market. Gradually, however, pills which released potassium more slowly and less catastrophically were developed. Careful clinical trials of the original preparation might have identified the frequent occurrence of gastric distress associated with them, even if they had missed the much rarer serious side effects.

Tonsillectomy and Adenoidectomy

Almost an entire generation of Americans had a set of their natural organs removed surgically, not because there was any particular need for the surgery, but simply because it became medically fashionable to perform it. No clinical trial has ever demonstrated that tonsils and adenoids should be removed in the absence of a few specific indications for the procedure. No benefits have ever been identified that outweigh the risks of exposing children (and adults, for that matter) to the risks of surgery where no serious problem existed. Tonsils and adenoids in children are larger than they are in adults, and they do tend to become involved in respiratory infections of childhood. Certainly, there are children who have special difficulties with these organs, including repeated infections that may lead to hearing problems through secondary infections involving the ear canals. Most children, though, have no greater trouble with their tonsils than an occasional sore throat. By the time they are fourteen or fifteen years old, the tonsils begin to shrink down and, as a rule, cause little problem from then on.

Persistent questions, as yet unanswered, remain with respect to the fact that the tonsils may play an important role in our immune systems and that removing them may be deleterious to health. This has been slowly recognized—though still without clinical proof in either direction—and the practice of removal has been tapering off over the past ten to fifteen years.

The list of abandoned medical therapies is long and will continue to grow. I recommend an interesting and popularly written book entitled *Modern Medical Mistakes*, which summarizes quite a lot of them.[1]

CURRENT PRACTICES ABOUT
WHICH THERE ARE DOUBTS

Many current medical practices are of questionable efficacy. The data in some cases are sufficient to indicate that the practice is simply not beneficial or, in some cases, is harmful.

Clofibrate to Prevent Heart Disease

Clofibrate is a drug which slightly lowers the level of cholesterol in the blood stream. Cholesterol, of course, plays a central
role in the development of heart disease and stroke. High levels
of blood cholesterol are associated with high rates of disease.
Therefore, it seems logical that anything which lowers the level
of cholesterol ought to contribute to a reduction in heart disease.
Clofibrate, estrogen (a female hormone), dextrothyroxine (a
thyroid drug), and niacin (a vitamin), are all known to reduce
serum cholesterol concentrations in the laboratory. In order to
determine whether these drugs could be given on a long-term
basis to reduce coronary heart disease while causing no serious
side effects, a nationwide, collaborative clinical trial was conducted in which persons with one or more previous heart attacks were randomly assigned to one of the above drugs or a
placebo. No one, including the study staff, knew who was taking which drug. Drugs were supplied under coded numbers,
and a break in the code occurred only in the case of medical
necessity.

Two of the drugs, dextrothyroxine and estrogen, were dis-
continued before the trial ended because persons taking them
had a significantly increased number of heart attacks. Significant side effects, not sufficient to stop the trial, occurred for all
the active drugs. Both clofibrate and niacin reduced serum
cholesterols compared to placebo, but the reduction was not
great. The effect of niacin was greater than that of clofibrate.
At the end of the trial the average period of observation for
each individual was more than six years. There was no difference in mortality or heart disease rates in the clofibrate, niacin,
or placebo groups.[2]

End of clofibrate and niacin? Not really. Three issues had to
be considered. First, the trial involved only persons with existing
heart disease, said some (including the clofibrate manufacturers), and it may work only on persons who have healthy systems with high cholesterol levels to begin with. Second, niacin,
while more effective than clofibrate at reducing heart disease,

had more unwanted side effects. Third, niacin was not under patent; clofibrate was. Therefore, enthusiasm for niacin waned, but clofibrate was sold with more vigor than ever. Now the ads showed diseased arteries and faces twisted in pain, and the copy told about reducing cholesterol (rather than heart disease). In tiny print detectable with the low-power lens of a microscope, these ads noted that clofibrate had not been shown to reduce coronary heart disease. But the total implication of these ads was precisely the opposite. Millions of patients have to contend with the costs and side effects of this well-tested but unproven drug, and doctors, too busy to deal with the frustrations of getting patients to change their diets, continue to prescribe it.

The British mounted another trial, this one involving healthy people with high, medium, and low cholesterol levels. They observed 15,745 men for an average of 5.3 years each. They achieved the same reduction in serum cholesterol level observed in the coronary drug project. They did observe a reduction in nonfatal heart attacks among the subgroup of men with the highest cholesterol levels, but there was no difference in fatal heart attacks. However, they also observed a significant *increase* in the total death rate among clofibrate-treated persons, primarily due to an excess of deaths related to the liver, biliary, and intestinal systems (all systems affected by the drug). They concluded that "the results of the trial confirm the basic hypothesis that reduction of high serum cholesterol levels, even in middle age, can reduce the incidence of IHD (ischemic heart disease). However, the fact that clofibrate increases the incidence of gallstones, and the possibility that it may have even more serious local pathological consequences, indicate that it cannot be recommended as a lipid-lowering drug for communitywide primary prevention of ischemic heart disease."[3]

Probably no drug has ever been more thoroughly or expensively tested than clofibrate. The fact that it is still prescribed widely, advertised extensively, and remains highly profitable for its manufacturer is a strong indication that evaluation alone is not sufficient to assure the adoption of wise medical practice.

At least two critical points in the determination of medical practice are inadequate in our current system. The first of these, as previously discussed, is evaluation. The second involves the translation of the findings of good evaluation into standard practice. Physicians are not trained in the evaluation of what they read, and the medical literature is as full of misinformation as the tabloid press. Physicians are trained to criticize whatever contradicts their training. This combination makes it difficult to transfer the findings of evaluation research into common practice.

Coronary Care Units

Most people who die from a heart attack are victims of disturbances in the electrical conduction of the heart muscle rather than of direct damage to the heart from the seizure. Technically, a heart attack is termed a myocardial infarction, or MI. Myocardial refers to heart muscle; infarction means the death of tissue as a result of insufficient blood (oxygen) supply to that tissue. After an MI, the heart is susceptible to fibrillation, a condition in which the normal synchronized contraction of heart muscle becomes chaotic and disorganized, resulting in the loss of effective pumping of blood. When this occurs, death follows rapidly unless the normal conduction patterns are quickly reestablished. It has long been known that a sudden electrical shock administered to the chest ("defibrillation") will often initiate normal heart-beats in someone who is undergoing fibrillation. In the meantime, while the defibrillator is being set up, appropriately applied pressure to the chest combined with ventilation of the lungs (cardiopulmonary resuscitation) can maintain life.

This knowledge was available by the early 1960s, and it was reasoned that someone who was undergoing a myocardial infarction would benefit from continuous observation where lifesaving measures might be instituted as soon as the need arose.

In addition, there were drugs that could suppress the kinds of abnormal beats which often preceded the onset of fibrillation. Continuous electrocardiographic monitoring could identify these beats before fibrillation occurred, and the drugs could be administered to prevent it. Special units were gradually established in various hospitals, and claims about their efficacy began appearing in the medical literature. They were not easy to refute. People who had suffered cardiac arrests and survived began to walk out of the hospitals. There was no doubt that if such arrests had taken place at home or, probably, even in a standard hospital ward, these people would not have survived.

In 1967 a classic study appeared which described the experience with coronary care units (CCUs) to date.[4] This paper was influential, despite the fact that no controlled, randomized studies of coronary care units had been performed. It led to a national conference on the subject in 1968, sponsored by the Department of Health, Education and Welfare. The conference proceedings clearly stated that efficacy of these units had not been demonstrated. Nevertheless, it was decided that, given the current level of information, such trials would not now be "ethically acceptable." A set of guidelines for coronary care units was published by the same agency that year, and CCUs proliferated rapidly in the ensuing few years. Despite the flood of "studies" purporting to show the benefits of these very expensive units, critics continued to point out that the "before/after" nature of these investigations was filled with uncontrollable bias and that not one of these studies had adequate control groups.

A group of investigators in England was especially interested in this question and worked hard, against a highly skeptical group of cardiologists, to obtain permission to do a truly randomized clinical trial. A. L. Cochrane, a brilliant and salty epidemiologist, is fond of describing the following story about how the trial first got underway. The decision was to randomly allocate persons who had undergone a myocardial infarction within

the preceding forty-eight hours, and who had no serious complications, to home or hospital care. The investigators were required to make a monthly report to the cardiologists so that the
trial could be stopped the moment it became evident that one
group had a significantly worse experience than the other.

Cochrane made the first of these reports. He announced that
more than forty persons had been randomized to each group
and that there had been twelve deaths among the home-care
group and eight among the hospital group. This information
was greeted with immediate demands to stop the trial, since the
death rate at home was 50 percent higher than the death rate
in the hospital. Cochrane regained the floor and reminded the
group that this difference was not statistically significant. That
is, with these small numbers, this difference might easily be observed by chance alone. The physicians were not mollified by
this statistical wizardry and continued to demand that the trial
be halted. Finally, Cochrane, no doubt with a slight grin on his
face, confessed that he had switched the numbers. There had
actually been eight deaths in the home-care group and twelve in
the hospital group. At that point, everyone agreed that these
results were not statistically significant and the trial should
proceed.

Eventually, the results indicated no difference in survival
after one year between home-treated and hospital-treated cases.
The home-treated group did slightly better initially.[5]

How can this be? If patients who have a cardiac arrest in a
CCU can be resuscitated, how can home care be as good? There
are two answers to this question. First, after a heart attack, the
heart is very sensitive to stress and anxiety, which seems to increase the likelihood of a cardiac arrest. A coronary care unit
can be an anxiety-provoking environment. Even the best of
them provides constant reminders to the patient of his or her
condition and separates the individual from normal, familiar
surroundings. The worst of them can be a nightmare, a place
where a sick person can hear the bleeping of his heart monitor,

see the desperate, even violent, attempts to revive other patients who have suffered an arrest, feel alone and separated from those who bring comfort, be bored to distraction by the fact that there is nothing to do (because, ironically enough, the stimulation of reading or television is regarded by some as being too excessive). Thus, while chances of survival are greater if heart arrest occurs in the CCU than at home, the chance of having the arrest in the first place may be greater in the CCU than at home. Second, persons who have an arrest are far more likely to have a second event at a later time, after they are out of the hospital. The fact that someone has been revived does not necessarily mean he has a long and productive life to live, although this does occur on occasion.

This first randomized trial of home treatment for heart attack was repeated by another group of British investigators who found precisely the same results: for the majority of persons who suffer a myocardial infarction, hospital care, despite its expense, "confers no clear advantage."[6] A retrospective review by a group of American investigators examined the methodological problems of previous studies and discussed potential sources of bias. Attempting to the degree possible to control for such bias, they found that death rates in CCU patients were twice as high as those not treated in CCUs.[7] They concluded that further randomized, controlled studies would be essential to determine which components of CCUs produce benefit, if any. Since cost of medical care is becoming an issue of increasing importance, and CCUs are so expensive, this is a critical subject for research.

My reason for discussing this issue in such depth is that, despite these findings, no serious consideration or even discussion of the role of the CCU in treating heart attack has been undertaken in this country. The drama of a cardiac resuscitation overwhelms the evidence that it might not have happened outside the CCU, and the existence of "community standards of practice" in the legal sense prohibits the formal evaluation in the United States of that practice, or its discontinuance, based on studies done in other countries. Hospitals rely on the income

CCUs generate; physicians and allied medical care personnel do too. The motivation to change on the basis of new knowledge is simply absent from the total organization.

Elective Hysterectomy

According to the National Center for Health Statistics, there were about 690,000 hysterectomies performed in the United States in 1973. At this rate, more than half the women in the population will have their uterus surgically removed before they reach age sixty-five. The probability that a woman will receive a hysterectomy varies enormously from place to place. Hysterectomy rates in the United States and Canada are more than double those in Great Britain. Within this country, there are two- to three-fold differences within different areas of the same state. As a medical student and later as an intern while working on gynecologic services, I was told by attending physicians that a woman past menopause had no further need of her uterus and that it might as well be removed to prevent the chance of developing cancer. On both occasions, my suggestion that the doctor might want to have his testicles cut off for the same reason was met with a disgusted and horrified look.

The indications for hysterectomy include cancer, benign tumors, chronic inflammation, disease of the supporting structures (which are usually late effects of childbirth), uterine involvement in other diseases of the pelvis, and major obstetrical complications, such as uncontrollable bleeding and rupture. These conditions may involve the vagina, cervix, ovaries, fallopian tubes, or uterus. However, many women have had hysterectomies because of what might be called "marginal" indications, including irregular menses, debilitating menstruation, profuse menstrual bleeding not sufficient to be life-endangering, and fear of pregnancy. In such cases hysterectomy becomes elective, resulting not from a life-threatening condition, but rather from one which makes life less comfortable.

An attempt has been made to analyze the costs and benefits of elective hysterectomy.[8] The investigators concluded that the "effect of hysterectomy on the life expectancy of a forty-year-old woman in good general health is small and uncertain, but appears to be slightly favorable." They indicated that the procedure could lead to relief of symptoms and consequent improved quality of life, but that there are "a good many potential unpleasant side effects associated with this operation" to balance that. Many of these are physical, but the more serious ones are related to mood and psyche. Depression requiring psychiatric intervention is not an uncommon result of hysterectomy, and many more women have psychologic difficulties that do not come to therapy. It is obvious that there are no ultimate answers to the question of whether or not elective hysterectomy is justifiable. Only an individual woman can make that decision, and few people can fully know in advance how they will be affected by the surgery. Nevertheless, it is disturbing to note that the best predictor of how many hysterectomies are carried out in any given region is the number of surgical specialists in the area. It is a consequence of the structure of our medical care system that incentives are provided to individual physicians to provide more care in their specialty areas. Nations which lack these incentives perform fewer surgeries. As the authors of the above study concluded:

> There are no data on what proportion of women, on the balance, are benefited by elective hysterectomy. While the benefits are unmeasured and uncertain, the costs are large. These costs are rarely paid by the patient. Society, if it is to pay the costs, must decide whether to allocate public funds for a procedure if it appears to be more of a convenience or luxury than a necessity.

OVERVIEW

In this chapter an attempt has been made to demonstrate that many medical therapies have been inadequately evaluated, that others which have been shown to be worthless continue to be used, and that still others are probably overused and of questionable value despite their enormous costs. In most instances it is not possible to make decisions about efficacy with absolute assurance. Therefore, it becomes necessary to make judgments based on the weight of evidence, keeping in mind that, in a world of limited resources, the decision to do something always involves the converse decision *not* to do something else. Recently, a physician wrote a letter to the *New England Journal of Medicine* criticizing that publication for printing an article on cost-benefit analysis of medical practice on the grounds that, where life is concerned, the only ethical thing to do is to do everything possible. Unfortunately, we cannot afford to do everything possible. Consequently, the only ethical thing left to do is to ask how to get the "best bang for the buck."

Chapter 9
Medical Care and the
Public Health

Comparing Turnips
to Oil Filters

*If you need to be sure
which way is right, you
can tell by their laughing
at it.*

—Lao Tzu

In the nineteenth century, Jules
Verne wrote a novel about going to
the moon in a balloon. Some have
considered this book remarkably
prescient, but the truth is that no
balloon, no matter how techno-
logically sophisticated, will ever
get anyone to the moon. In order
to get there it is necessary to scrap
the entire concept of transportation
that Verne used. If scientists of
subsequent times had said to themselves, "Aha, Jules Verne has
shown us how to get to the moon.
Let's solve the technical problems,"
we would not now have moon
rocks in our museums.

There are times when it is
necessary to examine the basic
conceptions which underlie the
scientific, social, political, and
economic norms under which we

operate. Such times are marked by upheaval and sometimes revolution, depending on how threatening a change of concept is to those in power and how strong the need for such a change. Galileo was hauled before the Inquisition for accurately reporting what he saw, a finding which cast doubt on the fundamental religious notion that man stood at the center of the universe. Martin Luther King was repeatedly jailed and was the subject of a campaign of slander by the FBI because he questioned the morality of segregation and dared to act, even though nonviolently, against it.

The brilliant and innovative leaders of the Revolutionary War, architects of the United States Constitution, were condemned criminals who would have been executed by the British if their revolution had failed. Their crime was, in principle, wanting to change a system. The Soviet Union has a long and illustrious record of suppressing dissent, but so, too, does nearly every other organized and powerful nation and group.

How does this relate to health? As I have already said, health and individual medical care are generally and mistakenly thought to be synonymous. This is largely because of the awesome image projected by medical care, a result of its role in the control of infectious diseases, advances in surgical techniques, and the development of new drugs. The degree to which these things contribute to improvements in health may be debated, but that they do contribute something cannot be argued. Further, they are dramatic, as demonstrated by the plethora of medical shows on television, medical novels, and the public's general fascination with medical information. This powerful image is reinforced by the vast expenditures on drug advertising and the almost reverent awe which many people have for physicians. The costs of that medical care system reflect the importance it has. In 1980 the United States health care industry made expenditures of some $200 billion, or nearly $1,000 for every individual in the nation.

THE GAP BETWEEN
CAUSE AND CARE

In 1974 the Canadian Ministry of National Health and Welfare published a document entitled *A New Perspective on the Health of Canadians*.[1] Lester Breslow, former dean of the School of Public Health at the University of California in Los Angeles, has termed this "the most significant health document of the twentieth century." It is a brief examination of the fundamental concepts underlying traditional notions of health care. For this reason it is highly threatening and widely ignored. Further, it is clearly written and comprehensible to any moderately literate person. (That a government agency managed to produce a comprehensible document is something of a mystery in itself!)

The document, which I shall refer to as the Canadian Health Plan, begins by quoting Thomas McKeown's assessment of the level of health in England and Wales from the eighteenth to the twentieth centuries.

In order of importance the major contributions to improvements in health in England and Wales were from limitation in family size (a behavioural change), increase in food supplies and a healthier physical environment (environmental influences), and specific preventive and therapeutic measures. . . .

Past improvement has been due mainly to modification of behaviour and changes in the environment and it is to these same influences that we must look particularly for further advance.[2]

Figure 9.1 presents trends in death rates in the United States for eight leading causes of death. A review of these major health problems with respect to the potential for decreasing the death rates is highly instructive.

1. Diseases of the heart. This is by far the leading class of

FIGURE 9.1
Age-Adjusted Death Rates for Selected Causes of Death, by Race:
United States, Selected Years 1950–1977

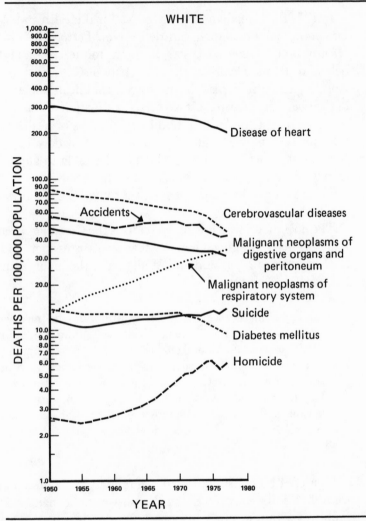

SOURCE: U.S. Department of Health, Education, and Welfare, *Health United States, 1979.* DHEW Publication No. (PHS) 80-1232, Washington, D.C., 1979. (Source: Division of Vital Statistics, National Center for Health Statistics, Unpublished data.)

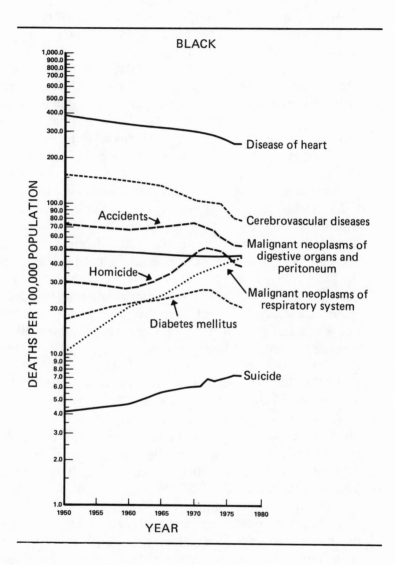

BLACK

DEATHS PER 100,000 POPULATION

Disease of heart

Cerebrovascular diseases

Accidents

Malignant neoplasms of digestive organs and peritoneum

Homicide

Malignant neoplasms of respiratory system

Diabetes mellitus

Suicide

YEAR

fatal illness. There has been a slight but significant decline in death rate from these diseases in the past ten to fifteen years. This decline accounted for primarily by a reduction in new cases, not by improved longevity for those who have already developed the disease. Many mysteries still surround the causes of heart disease, as has been previously discussed, but it is clearly related to environment. Diet plays a role. So do cigarette smoking, stress and personality type, heredity, and other factors. Most important, the majority of persons who die of a heart attack do so *before* they reach medical care. Thus, all of the therapeutic knowledge in the universe could not prevent the majority of these deaths. Simple preventive measures can.

2. Cerebrovascular diseases. The physiologic mechanisms which lead to a heart attack are similar to those which produce stroke. In stroke, an area of the brain is deprived of oxygen as a result of a hemorrhage or a blockage of a blood vessel. When the brain cells die, the functions associated with that area of the brain are lost. If the affected region is large enough, death results. Generally, those risk factors associated with stroke are not too different from those leading to heart attack. Blood pressure is somewhat more important; cholesterol somewhat less. Blood pressure, though, is affected in part by the level of salt in the diet and by weight. A fat person with a high salt diet and resulting high blood pressure is a likely candidate for a stroke. As with heart disease, most persons who die of stroke do so before they reach medical care. Therapeutic measures for treating stroke are very limited, and are primarily directed to rehabilitation of function after the danger of death has passed. The potential for reducing the death rate from stroke through medical treatment is limited.

3. Accidents. Because accidents are not caused by germs, and because they strike suddenly rather than slowly, they are often thought of as freak occurrences, a piece of bad luck that always happens to the other guy. In fact, as figure 9.1 makes clear, accidents kill more people than lung or digestive cancers, the lead-

ing forms of malignancy. More important, accidents kill the young more often than the old. Table 9.1 is taken from the Canadian Health Plan and presents the years of life lost to various major causes of death in Canada. This figure, referred to in

TABLE 9.1
Years of Life Lost to Various Causes of Death in Canada

Cause	Years Lost— Male	Years Lost— Female
Motor vehicle accidents	154,000	59,000
Ischemic heart disease	157,000	36,000
All other accidents	136,000	43,000
Respiratory disease and lung cancer	90,000	50,000
Suicide	51,000	18,000
Total	588,000	206,000

SOURCE: Adapted from M. Lalonde, *A New Perspective on the Health of Canadians. A Working Document.* Ottawa: Ministry of National Health and Welfare, 1974.

previous chapters, is calculated by multiplying the number of deaths times the average number of years of life lost by a person dying of the given cause. That is, if an individual dies at age thirty, he loses more than forty years of life, but if he dies at age sixty-five he loses only a few years. Using this criterion, automobile accidents *alone* are the single greatest cause of lost years of life—worse than heart disease, cancer, or stroke. Automobile safety legislation and the construction of safe roads, therefore, are issues of major health significance. Improved trauma units and emergency rooms may save a few more accident victims, but they do not address the problem in any meaningful or basic way. It is possible to argue that automobile safety is our number one health problem.

4. Respiratory cancer. Respiratory cancers were rare until cigarette smoking became popular in the twentieth century. Since then, they have become the leading cause of cancer deaths. Men started smoking before women and, therefore, ex-

perienced an early rise in lung cancer deaths. By the end of World War II, women were taking up smoking in increasing numbers; about fifteen years later the rates of lung cancer in women began to skyrocket. Today smoking has declined slightly among men and so has the rate of lung cancer. But women are smoking more than ever, and soon lung cancer deaths in women may exceed those in men. The treatment of lung cancer has changed little in the past forty years. The chance of living five years after the initial diagnosis is still less than 5 percent. Opportunities to treat the disease are minimal. Prevention is as simple—and as complex—as not smoking.

5. Malignant neoplasms of digestive organs and peritoneum. This includes cancers of the entire digestive tract and the peritoneum which surrounds the abdominal organs. The colon is the commonest site for cancers in this category, but they may occur anywhere in the entire digestive tract. Less is known about the causes of these cancers than about the other conditions being considered here. There is some evidence that colon cancer occurs more often in persons who eat highly refined, low-fiber diets which are common in industrialized nations. Medical treatment of these cancers has improved over the last few decades, and this is probably responsible for the slight decline in death rates seen in figure 9.1. The potential for prevention in this area is unclear. Some think that most colon cancer would disappear if we ate a diet high in fiber and low in fat, but this contention is unproven. Dramatic changes in rates of cancer may occur without the faintest hint as to why. The rapid decline in stomach cancer discussed earlier is an example.

6. Suicide. Clearly, medical treatment of attempted suicide victims is not a viable means for dealing with the problem. Although lives are saved through prompt, effective medical therapy, this therapy does not deal with the factors which led to the suicide attempt in the first place or with preventing another attempt. In this way, suicide is no different from heart disease or cancer. Medical treatment does not address cause or

prevention. Persons who have a single heart attack or who survive the removal of a cancer are still at vastly increased risk of a second similar event just as persons who attempt suicide are likely to do so again unless the basic depression which led to the attempt is dealt with.

7. Diabetes mellitus. Often termed "sugar diabetes," this is a condition in which medical treatment has clearly been successful in prolonging life. This is particularly true for the more severe diabetics who are dependent on daily insulin injections. Medical therapies have been largely unsuccessful in dealing with the long-term vascular and neurologic effects of diabetes, although exciting new discoveries may soon change this picture. At first glance it may seem that public health and preventive medicine can accomplish little in this area, although it is possible that weight control might prevent the development of the milder form of adult-onset diabetes. This view is somewhat misleading, however. Diabetics are particularly susceptible to cardiovascular disease, and for them it is even more important to control the other factors which lead to such illnesses. Diabetics are usually told to avoid sugar because sweets may precipitate an acute diabetic attack, but they are usually not told to avoid cigarette smoking or informed of the critical importance of a low fat diet and control of blood pressure. A glance at a diabetic dinner plate in your local hospital will confirm this assertion. Yet, everything known about heart disease points to the additive, sometimes multiplicative, nature of various risk factors. If you have one, it becomes that much more important to avoid the others. We can't prevent diabetes directly, nor can we cure it. We can reduce the long-term consequences by applying the same wisdom to those consequences that would be applied to nondiabetics.

8. Homicide. The most startling piece of information in figure 9.1 is the homicide curve. The number of homicides is increasing rapidly. Among blacks as of 1977, respiratory cancers, digestive cancers, and murder all take approximately the same

number of lives. Roughly twice as many blacks are murdered as die of diabetes; more are murdered than die of influenza, pneumonia, or cirrhosis. More whites and blacks are murdered than die of tuberculosis, arteriosclerosis, bronchitis, emphysema, asthma, cystic fibrosis, multiple sclerosis, or any of countless other conditions for which well-meaning foundations and enormous public interest exist. But the medical care system, the legislative structure, and the legal enforcement apparatus do not deal with the escalating violence except in a superficial "treatment" oriented manner.

The reason for presenting these nine conditions as examples is to demonstrate that the existing systems for dealing with health issues have no mechanism for attempting to mitigate problems. In a sense, the medical care system is to the public health problem what aspirin is to a brain tumor. Relief of symptoms is not an answer, and treatment of an individual does nothing to stop the spread of disease to others or its recurrence in the same individual. Once again, let me emphasize that this is *not* to say that the medical care system is useless or that it fails to help people who are sick. It does these things and does them well. If I had symptoms of serious illness, I would go quickly to a physician's office for examination and, if need be, treatment. But that treatment, no matter how successful, would not deal with what made me sick in the first place nor would it prevent a recurrence of the same or of some other illness.

The Canadian Health Plan arrived at a similar conclusion, and its authors decided that a solution was to completely change the way we view health and illness.

THE HEALTH FIELD CONCEPT

By examining the causes and underlying factors which produce illness and death, the authors of the Canadian Health Plan identified four major areas which contribute to ill health. They concluded that each of these four areas required attention in order to maximize the health status of the population.

1. Human biology. This area includes all aspects of mental and physical health which occur as a consequence of the physiological and genetic makeup of an individual. It includes heredity, aging, the optimal functioning of internal organ systems, mental retardation, and congenital malformations.

2. Environment. This category consists of health matters that are external to the body and over which the individual has little or no control. The safety of food, drugs, water, air, and consumer products all fall into this area. So, too, do sewage disposal, safety in the workplace, and control of the spread of communicable diseases.

3. Lifestyle. This category includes all personal decisions made by individuals which have a bearing on health. Many people have ways of living which are clearly deleterious to health, and these habits or decisions have become an integral and important part of their lives. Factors in this area include cigarette smoking, obesity, drug abuse (including alcoholism), insufficient exercise, nonnutritious diets, and reckless driving.

4. Health care organization. This area includes what we traditionally think of as medical care. At the present time, the vast majority of health resources are expended in this category. It includes the quantity, quality, arrangement, nature, and relationships of people and resources in the provision of health care.

The imbalance of attention to these areas is demonstrated in table 9.2 in which expenditures by Canada in each of the four areas are compared along with the changes over time from 1969 to 1974. For every $1.00 spent on environmental health problems in 1973–74, $1.04 was spent on human biology, $1.18 on lifestyle, and $60.43 on health care organization. In the United States, priorities are quite similar, although per capita expenditures on health care organization are even greater. In fact, it is

TABLE 9.2
Health Expenditures in Canada by Health Field
Fiscal Years 1969–70 and 1973–74

1. DISTRIBUTION ($ MILLIONS)

Year	Human Biology	Environment	Life-style	Health Care Organization
1969–70	31.2	21.5	12.0	1,255.8
1970–71	34.4	24.2	12.7	1,552.1
1971–72	36.1	26.3	23.3	1,903.2
1972–73	38.1	34.9	28.9	2,095.5
1973–74	40.1	38.4	45.4	2,320.4

2. PERCENTAGE AND DOLLAR INCREASE 1969–70 TO 1973–74

	Percentage	$ Millions
Human biology	29	8.9
Environment	79	16.9
Life-style	278	33.4
Health care organization	85	1,064.6

SOURCE: Adapted from M. Lalonde, *A New Perspective on the Health of Canadians. A Working Document.* Ottawa: Ministry of National Health and Welfare, 1974.

critical that people realize that the costs of medical care are rapidly approaching the point where society can no longer afford to finance them. As resources become increasingly limited, how do we choose between improved technology for the wealthy and improved access to care for the masses? This issue has been central in struggles over health care priorities in recent years. The noise and vituperation generated by the argument have obscured the essential fact that neither approach is optimal for improving the health of the nation. Both sides involve maintaining the lopsided level of expenditures directed to medical care.

Physicians are often aghast when I make this point. The medical problems of society are vast, they counter, and we have a long way to go toward providing adequate medical care. Can you be serious in saying that expenditures in this area should be cut in order to finance programs in the areas of lifestyle, environment, and human biology? Would you really use money that could be spent on a new surgical unit to push a health-related law through the legislature?

The choice is difficult, but the answer is clearly yes. If you were in a lifeboat between two sinking vessels, one with ten persons aboard, the other with one person aboard, and you only had time to save the occupants of one of the boats, you would clearly choose the one with ten passengers. This is precisely the issue we face in allocating health care resources.

MEDICAL CARE, DOLLARS, AND HEALTH

The same A. L. Cochrane who presented the reversed numbers of deaths for the coronary care unit study to a group of incredulous cardiologists (chapter 8) recently published a paper in which he and his co-workers examined the relationships between the amount of money spent on medical care in eighteen developed countries and the mortality rates in those nations.[3] They selected countries with equivalent soundness of statistical data for comparison. They also included some basic environmental and dietary factors to compare the relationship between these factors and mortality with that between medical care and mortality. The findings of this study are stunning in their implications.

1. *None* of the seven indices of available health services (numbers of doctors, nurses, acute hospital beds, pediatricians, obstetricians, midwives, and percent of gross national product spent on health) was negatively correlated with mortality in a consistent way. In all but one age group, the number of doctors per person was *positively* associated with the national mortality rate (i.e., the more doctors the higher the death rate).

2. The major factors associated with low death rates were,

in order of importance, gross national product per person, density of population, sugar consumption, and the percent of health care provided by public funds.

3. The major factors associated with high death rates were cigarette consumption, alcohol consumption, and numbers of doctors.

Please do not interpret the data to assume that everything which is associated with low or high death rates necessarily causes (or prevents) death. Nevertheless, for something to be causal, it must be statistically associated with the thing it is supposed to cause. Adjustment of the data above, for example, suggested that the association of sugar consumption with low death rates was not due to diet, but rather to other factors with which high sugar consumption is associated. Eating sugar will not improve your health. The important findings are the negative ones. Health care services are not related to low death rates; environmental and lifestyle factors are.

It follows, then, that spending as much money as we do on medical care is akin to the drunk looking for his wallet under a streetlight though he lost it in a nearby alley. When asked why he didn't look in the alley where he lost it, he replied that he could see better under the light.

QUALITY VERSUS QUANTITY

Because mortality is easy to measure, comparisons of the health status of different societies are usually presented, as they are above, in terms of mortality differences. Occasionally efforts will be made to compare differences in disease rates (morbidities), but this requires more effort and it limits the comparisons to those nations which keep comparable morbidity statistics. Health organizations and agencies seldom pay attention to the quality of life. The World Health Organization in its definition of health includes references to physical, mental and social well-being, but in practice, physical survival receives most of the attention and resources.

Yet, despite its steadily increasing life expectancy, the United States is not a pleasant place in which to grow old. Many of the elderly live below the poverty level; retirement is often forced rather than voluntary, and little use is made of the skills and energy of this group. The visible evidence of what awaits our final years is apt to take some of the edge from the keenness of our daily life. Instead of asking how we can live more satisfying, fulfilled lives, we have created institutions which ask only how we can live longer, and quality be damned. Strategies developed for promoting and maintaining health are of little use to society unless they consciously address the total concept of health embodied in that World Health Organization definition. This implies careful consideration of those things which contribute to well-being, and an understanding of what "well-being" actually is. This requires a further understanding of the differences between "normal" and "optimal" functioning. Earlier, I used the example of the difference between a "normal" and an "optimal" cholesterol in predicting risk of death from heart disease. Normal usually is defined by the average. But if an entire society is malfunctioning, then the average may be a misleading substitute for the optimal. The extreme levels of suicide and homicide in our society suggest that a fundamental examination of values might be in order.

STRATEGIES FOR IMPROVEMENT

The Canadian Health Plan outlined five strategies for improving health. Their implementation might differ, depending on the definition of health one accepts. As before, I use the definition of the World Health Organization. The five strategies are listed here.

A Health Promotion Strategy

Plans and programs must be designed to inform and assist people and organizations in adopting behaviors and accepting responsibility for personal matters relating to social, mental, and physical health. As with other strategies, complex ethical issues are raised in attempting to plan such programs. We are not islands, as John Donne noted centuries ago. Personal health behavior often affects others who take no direct part in the behavior. Drinking drivers kill sober drivers; smokers who die prematurely from the effects of cigarettes leave families behind. The greater the density of population, the more conflict there is between the opposing values. Thus, solutions that worked in the past may not work in the future. Nearly all large cities ban the backyard burning of trash; small cities do not. This is strictly a function of population density. The more people there are, the less freedom each can have.

A Regulatory Strategy

A clear role exists for legislative action in reducing health risks. Should there be standards for purity and safety in drugs and food? Of course, most of us would say. Standards for clean water and air? For the control of hazardous chemicals and radioactive wastes? What about controls on the degree to which we are exposed to commercial advertising that urges us to adopt certain behaviors, such as cigarette smoking? Currently, the tobacco companies in the United States spend in excess of $1 billion annually (nearly $5 for every person in the nation) convincing us to smoke cigarettes. That is freedom of speech, we are often told, but legislative efforts to counter this massive attempt at public brainwashing are usually viewed as governmental intrusions into personal lives. The notion that corporations with a profit motive are not intruding into our personal lives when they try to get us to do (or not do) something, but that government doing the same thing, is intruding, seems ludicrous to me. The solution is neither obvious nor easy, but the status quo has made cigarette-induced lung cancer the leading cause of cancer deaths.

A Research Strategy

Currently there is little coordination in our efforts to solve complex health problems. Money goes where it is fashionable to send it, without much sense of priority. It has become unacceptable in the last decade to spend much money on basic research into understanding the essentials of human biology. Instead, an emphasis has been placed on immediate results. But basic research provides the capital, and goal-directed research is the interest on that capital. The medical advances of the last decade have largely been made by spending existing capital without any reinvestment. There is not a great deal more in the way of immediate results that we can obtain from our depleted account of basic research.

A Health Care Efficiency Strategy

The organization of medical care leaves a lot to be desired. It is essentially a laissez-faire system in which all of the incentives are to provide more and more care, whether or not it is needed, at higher and higher costs. A national health insurance program that does not deal with the nature of these perverse incentives will not solve the financial crisis in health care.

A Goal-Setting Strategy

We must decide where we want to go. Then, we must plan the means to get there. Since resources are limited, this requires setting priorities and making some difficult decisions. It also involves stepping on lots of toes. The best means to minimize the opposition this will generate is to involve all interested parties in setting goals and making decisions on priorities.

Humankind has an inherent problem that could bring about

its extinction—unless we become alert to it. From the evolu-
tionary standpoint, the least specialized creatures are the ones
best able to adapt to changes in environment and, therefore, are
those least vulnerable to extinction. Humans, however, have become nonspecialized almost to the point of specialization. We
have become so adaptable that we are willing to accept too
much. Anyone from the countryside who has visited Los Angeles on a smoggy day is amazed that anyone will tolerate living
in such a place. But the natives all say that it's not really so bad
when you get used to it. We have forgotten, particularly in the
eastern part of the nation, what it was to swim and fish in the
rivers, and we accept it as the price of "progress." We are used
to pervasive noise—no city is ever silent, as becomes obvious the
moment it is left behind—and we have accepted an endless
sense of being rushed as the price of success and progress. We
have even learned to live with and ignore the fact that more
than fifty thousand nuclear weapons stand poised to destroy
the world we know. Our adaptability may, indeed, be our
downfall.

Solutions to the problems of health and well-being have not
emerged over the thousands of years of human civilization, and
they will not until conscious, directed effort is put into defining
goals and moving toward them. Better technology and more
hospitals and doctors won't get us there. Neither will boundless
optimism, nor hopeless pessimism, nor dull apathy.

To be healthy and well, we must be able to stand far enough
outside of our daily routines to determine what it is we are
doing to ourselves and how that relates to what we want for
ourselves.

Chapter 10
Some Current
Controversies

Why the Answer Is
Never the Solution

Epidemiology is a science which
has controversy as its major output.
It uses methods which are not well
understood by most other scientists
and which invite misinterpretation
by journalists and the public.
Recently the *New England Journal
of Medicine* published an article
linking coffee drinking and pancreatic cancer. This article received
extraordinary attention from the
press and public. Hysteria resulted,
and tens of thousands more made
that statement: "Why should I do
anything at all. Everything is bad
for me."

The publicity was unwarranted;
the defeatism it engendered was
unfortunate. The press has shown
a remarkable lack of understanding
of the implications of these studies.
This has resulted in some popular,

157

and thoroughly misinterpreted, reports of perfectly good scientific work. The study in question was a case-control study in which coffee-drinking histories were taken from persons with pancreatic cancer and also from a control group of persons with other conditions. In chapter 5 I discussed the uses and shortcomings of this kind of study. As you will recall, case-control studies are useful for forming hypotheses about questions which deserve more intensive study. Only under rather uncommon circumstances can they reasonably be used to infer cause and effect. Those uncommon circumstances include the existence of supporting data from laboratory and animal studies as well as a consistency of findings across several different populations. None of these circumstances was present in the coffee-pancreas story. The study was well performed by competent investigators. But it was a first and uncorroborated report. No animal information and no known underlying pathophysiologic mechanism are recognized to explain the observed relationship.

A reasonable response to the report would have been to follow the authors' suggestion that other researchers note the finding and begin seeking confirmatory evidence from their own data. If this evidence were forthcoming, other kinds of studies, especially prospective ones, might be conducted if feasible, or previous data sets, such as the Framingham study that include information on coffee drinking, might have been examined for a relation between coffee and pancreatic cancer. Animal studies might have been performed in which coffee was examined for effects on the pancreas, and tissue culture studies might also observe the potential mutagenicity of coffee. If such studies were in general agreement (not total, since no one ever agrees totally about anything), then cautious public press releases would be appropriate.

The misinterpretation of this report, however, was so extreme that one evening news program showed a large sign behind the announcer which proclaimed a relationship between caffeine and cancer. In fact, coffee contains many substances besides caffeine, and the published report did not discuss caffeine at all, except to point out that no such relationship was observed between tea drinking and pancreatic cancer. Since many teas also contain caffeine, caffeine is certainly not the most likely cause, even if a relationship between coffee and cancer does exist.

Given that epidemiologic methods must be used to search for health effects of environmental factors and behaviors, and that such methods contain a hierarchy of approaches ranging from observation of trends to formation of hypotheses to inference of cause, the potential for misunderstanding is great among persons who fail to understand that hierarchy. In the remainder of this chapter, I will deal with a few of the controversial areas in epidemiology and examine why they remain controversial.

DIET AND HEART DISEASE

The relationship between diet and heart disease has been alluded to throughout this book. There are two reasons for this. First, it is the area which perhaps best epitomizes epidemiologic controversy. Second, as a researcher and teacher of the epidemiology of cardiovascular diseases, I am most familiar with the details and background of the subject.

To review briefly, in the 1940s it was noted that human populations that have low fat, low cholesterol diets tend to have lower rates of heart disease than other cultures, although exceptions to this general rule have been identified. In the 1950s and 1960s it was repeatedly confirmed that persons free of heart disease who had high levels of blood cholesterol were much more likely to develop heart disease as time went on than were those with low cholesterol levels. It was also demonstrated that a diet high in saturated fats, which come largely from meat and meat products as well as solid vegetable shortenings, produced an increase in blood cholesterol. Animal studies indicated that the classic changes of cardiovascular disease could be induced in animals by the addition of saturated fats and cholesterol to the diet.

Because eggs constitute one of the few sources of cholesterol which does not also contain a high level of saturated fat, confusion emerged as to the relative roles of dietary saturated fat and dietary cholesterol in producing heart disease and in raising blood cholesterol. This confusion has not yet been resolved. It is clear that solid fats raise blood cholesterol, less clear that dietary cholesterol alone has this effect. Naturally, this small distinction has enormous industrial and economic implications. The egg industry wants exoneration of their product, and the National Livestock and Meat Board, which once referred to the medical director of the American Heart Association, Dr. Cambell Moses, as the "high priest of polyunsaturation," denies everything.

Studies further demonstrated that dietary reduction of fats could lead to a reduction in blood cholesterol levels in humans, just as they had in animals. A growing recognition of the fact that diet does not explain everything about heart disease also helped clarify the exceptions observed. Some people apparently are more genetically susceptible to a rise in blood cholesterol when they eat high fat diets. Other factors may also interact with diet to produce heart disease. Cigarettes, a competitive, stressful personality, and high blood pressure may be involved.

Just about the time that some agreement seemed to be emerging a controversial article appeared in the *New England Journal*.[1] This article is worth reading because it makes virtually every error of interpretation discussed in this book. It denies that diet substantially changes cholesterol levels, despite the fact that studies reporting such changes are widely available. It uses crude mortality rate trends to refute that changes in diet have led to a reduction in heart disease, despite extremely well-documented evidence of such a change. "Crude rate" means that changes in the age distribution of the population are not accounted for. Thus, as the average age of the population increases (which it is doing) crude death rates will rise, because there are more old people and they die more frequently than do young people. The death rates within any given age group for *heart disease* (Mann did not use death rates for heart disease, but rather for all causes) have clearly declined. Responses to the article were published several months later,[2] but the article remains widely quoted by those who have not examined it or considered the responses.

In 1980 the U.S. Department of Health and Human Services, which had been researching this issue for more than thirty years, finally issued dietary guidelines which included a recommendation that Americans eat less fat and less meat. At the same time, for reasons that are somewhat obscure, a special panel was formed by the National Research Council to recommend dietary guidelines. This panel, most of whose members had close ties to the food industry, failed to find convincing evidence that dietary fat or cholesterol should be reduced. The report was widely publicized, but the rationale for this conclusion was not. First, the panel decided to ignore all of the highly consistent animal study evidence because, after all, animals are not people. Second, they decided to ignore all of the epidemiologic evidence, also highly consistent, because the epidemiologic studies did not conform to Koch's postulates, a formal set of laboratory guidelines for determining the microorganisms responsible for a given infectious disease. (Of course it would be ethically impossible to perform any experiment on human beings in conformation with Koch's postulates.) Third, they decided to accept only human studies in which efforts to change diet had been made and the eventual effects on heart disease assessed. They identified five such studies, none of which suc-

ceeded in demonstrating a reduction in heart disease among
study subjects. This seems to prove the panel's conclusion until
you realize that none of these five studies could have demonstrated such a reduction!

In 1969 a national conference was held to determine whether
or not a large-scale study should be conducted to determine the
impact of a low-fat diet on reducing the future risk of heart
disease among high-risk persons. The conference decided that
such a study would require some forty thousand high-risk persons and would cost in excess of a billion dollars. This was regarded as not feasible. The decision about diet must be made
through indirect means—the concurrence of different lines of
research. The largest of the five studies cited by the National
Research Council had 571 persons, or slightly more than 1 percent of the number required to answer the question.

In the case of the diet-heart disease controversy, the dispute
is principally between researchers and industrial-political interests. There are genuine questions about the relative importance
of diet in relation to other factors, about the role of dietary
cholesterol apart from saturated fats, and about the degree to
which existing disease of the cardiovascular system might be
reversed by changes in the diet. There is little doubt, though,
that in spite of the smokescreen of criticism generated by the
food industry, diet does play a role in producing heart disease
and that most Americans would be better off eating less fat than
they do.

HEALTH RISKS OF OBESITY

Not infrequently, popular articles claim that being overweight isn't unhealthy after all. Such reports are usually based
on single studies which are seldom placed in the context of
the total research that has been performed on the subject. The
reasons that the relationships between obesity and various illnesses have been so confusing are only now becoming apparent.

They are summarized in a short article in the *British Medical Journal.*[3]

If human beings had designed the universe, all relationships would probably be linear. That is, when two factors are related to each other, a change in one factor would always be associated with the same degree of change in the other. For example, we might assume that there is a linear relationship between the numbers of animals in a herd and the food supply available, that a given level of food would always be associated with a given population. However, things were obviously not placed in the hands of a linear designer. Within certain limits, food and population are generally related, but if food supplies increase, population doesn't keep pace beyond a certain point. Other factors come into play, such as the amount of space available and the level of communicable diseases (which rises dramatically with overcrowding), and so on.

It is fair to say that obese people of both sexes have a tendency to die at an earlier age than their nonobese peers. Studies which appear to contradict this general statement are simply focused on a narrow piece of the relationship between excessive weight and health where the expected linear rules don't hold. Overweight is a significant predictor of death in persons under fifty to fifty-five years of age. Above that age, obesity does not predict an increase in death risk. A major portion of the relationship between obesity and risk of death is explained by the fact that fat people have, on the average, higher blood pressure, more diabetes, and higher blood cholesterol levels than lean people. In some studies this has been reported as indicating that obesity is not an "independent" risk factor. The media often interpret that statement as meaning that overweight is not a true cause of death or illness, but that is a misinterpretation of the findings. Lack of "independence" simply means that some of the effects of weight on health are explained by the fact that obesity raises blood pressure, cholesterol, and blood sugar. Losing weight lowers those factors and thereby probably contributes to improved health and reduced risk of dying. People who are extremely thin are often in poor health and will, if lumped with the lean but healthy, make that group appear to be less healthy than it really is. In other words, the relationship between weight and risk of death is *not* linear like this:

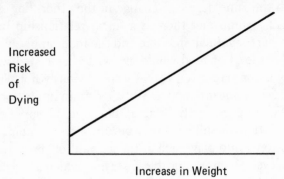

Increase in Weight

but rather, it is U-shaped, like this:

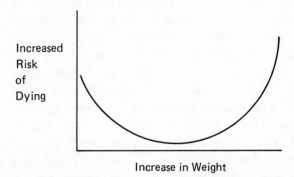

Increase in Weight

As the previously cited article concludes: "The nature of the link between overweight and excess mortality seems likely to have several components: inactivity and hyperlipidemia [high blood fats] . . . may be implicated, as may other factors such as the difficulty in providing medical care for obese people and their increased anaesthetic and surgical risks."

CAUSES OF CANCER

Perhaps no area of disease prevention has been subjected to more argument, public scrutiny, or regulatory and political infighting than the questions surrounding the causes and prevention of cancers. A bit of perspective is in order. First, cancer is not a single disease, but a multiplicity of conditions. We know from animal as well as human studies that some cancers are hereditary, some are caused by exposures to mutagenic chemicals, some by radiation, and still others by viruses. Obviously, it is inappropriate to talk about "the" cause of cancer, since many such causes exist. Second, susceptibility to cancer-producing agents appears to be highly dependent on the status of the individual immune systems of persons exposed to causal factors as well as to the total degree of exposure which has occurred. Think of your immune system as a dam which may be large or small. The function of this dam is to hold back the "flood" of disease. A small dam can prevent a small flood, but not a large one. The larger the dam, the more exposure can be tolerated before disease occurs. This analogy is applicable to most diseases, not just to cancer.

The controversies surrounding cancer and its causes center, as do many health controversies, over differences in philosophies more than in scientific evidence. This is a crucial distinction, because no discussion of philosophy can have a satisfactory outcome when it is based on scientific evidence. Yet, this is precisely what occurs in both government and industry. But a little more background is in order before discussing that issue.

A review of animal research clearly demonstrates that the occurrence of cancer in animals can be influenced by physical and psychological variations in the environment.[4] Such things as excessive handling, isolation, electric shock, surgical wounds, early weaning, and exercise have been shown to influence the occurrence and/or course of various tumors. The nature of the association is not clear. There may be critical periods and circumstances when certain manipulations are harmful, manipulations which are not otherwise deleterious. Human studies have also indicated frequent but inconsistent relationships between cancer and periods of stress, both mental and physical. The nature of these relationships is not at all defined. Some popular press articles claim that depressed people get more cancers than nondepressed people. It isn't that simple. The following list summarizes general factors now recognized to be associated with cancer.

1. Heredity
2. Mutagenic chemicals, substances (e.g., tobacco tar, polyvinyl chloride, etc.)
3. Radiation
4. Viruses (role in humans unclear, but highly likely)
5. Psychological and physical environments (e.g., "stress." Nature of relationships not clear)

A second line of evidence for the environmental and behavioral influences on cancer concerns cross-cultural comparisons. Table 10.1 is taken from an article by a distinguished British cancer epidemiologist, Richard Doll.[5] It presents the highest and lowest rates of occurrence for various common cancers in different cultures. Cancer of the esophagus, for example, has a three hundred-fold range of incidence. That is, in northeast Iran it is three hundred times more common than it is in Nigeria, and breast cancer is seven times more common in Connecticut than it is in Uganda. When natives of one culture move to another culture, they gradually assume the cancer rates of the adopted culture, demonstrating that these are not genetic or racial differences, but environmental ones.

Large changes in the occurrences of various cancers within a given culture may occur over time. I have already discussed the decline in cancer of the stomach which has occurred in the

TABLE 10.1
Common Cancers: Approximate Range of Variation of
Cumulative Incidence Rates up to Seventy-five Years of Age

Cancer Site	Approximate Range of Variation	High Incidence Area	Risk %	Low Incidence Area	Risk %
Esophagus	X 300	Northeast Iran	20	Nigeria	0.1
Skin	X 150	U.S.A., Texas, white	17	India, Bombay	0.1
Bronchus	X 100	England	11	Nigeria	0.1
Stomach	X 50	Japan	11	Uganda	0.2
Cervix uteri	X 20	Colombia	10	Israel, Jewish	0.6
Liver	X 70	Mozambique	8	Norway	0.1
Prostate	X 20	U.S.A., black	7	Japan	0.3
Breast	X 7	U.S.A., Connecticut	7	Uganda	0.9

SOURCE: Adapted from R. Doll, "Epidemiology of Cancer: Current Perspectives," *American Journal of Epidemiology* 104 (1976): 397. Reprinted with the permission of the author and publisher.

United States since the 1940s. These cultural differences and time changes provide a handle for grasping the problems of cancer prevention. As Doll says, epidemiologic studies have pointed the way for prevention and helped define those environmental conditions responsible for the production of disease.

Table 10.2, also from Doll, presents some known occupational cancers and their associated causes. Of the twenty exposures listed here which are known to produce cancer in persons excessively exposed, only three were first identified by animal studies. The others were detected using epidemiologic approaches which confirmed higher rates for the indicated cancers among persons exposed to chemicals than among persons not exposed. In the case of nasal sinus cancer among leather workers and hardwood furniture makers, the specific agent has not been identified. Without the opportunity to obtain medical information on thousands of exposed and unexposed workers, the risks of these substances and the opportunity to take protective measures would not have been recognized.

This brief and incomplete list of carcinogenic agents raises that philosophical issue I mentioned earlier. Regulatory bodies are caught in a dilemma. On the one hand, they are charged with protecting the welfare of the public; on the other, they must not impede progress which will benefit the public. These two worthy goals are in direct conflict. Whether the issue is a new drug, the use of a new chemical in industry, a food additive to prevent spoilage, or the release of a waste product into water or air, there is a conflict between the need to protect those exposed and the need to develop technologies that will improve the general well-being.

No scientific study can ever prove that something is *not* harmful. It can only conclude that, given the study conditions, the limitations of sample size, and duration of follow-up, no harmful effects were observed. Large effects which occur immediately are easily detected. Small effects which require years to surface are nearly impossible to detect prior to regulatory approval. Because cancer is a rare outcome (that is, it occurs in only a small fraction of the population in any given year), and because its effects may occur only after years of exposure, the determination that a given chemical produces cancer *cannot* be made in any study that is financially and temporally feasible prior to general use. It is crucial that the public recognize this.

Testing of drugs and chemical exposures on humans detects only the largest and most immediate of effects prior to such approval. It is impossible to do otherwise. The assumption that this approval represents a certainty that the substance in question is safe in the long run is totally fallacious. Further, such testing invariably involves only the single substance in question. In real life, workers and the general public are exposed to a number of new and uncertain substances whose combined effects are completely unknown and will remain unknown. We are, for example, exposed to several hundred different food additives, many of which produce mutagenic changes in laboratory testing. No human effects have been observed for these compounds tested singly for short periods of time in small numbers of people. But that is not how they are used in the real world. Unraveling the effects of three of these substances which interact to produce disease only in men of oriental background under age 50, for example, is simply not possible.

It seems to me that this reality ought to suggest some policy guidelines. If a substance contributes substantially to public well-being, it may be worth a small risk of long-term harm. But why should we take chances with chemicals, such as food colorings, which accomplish nothing but to reinforce distorted notions of what food ought to look like? If you make your own potato chips at home, they will appear too white. What is wrong with them? They lack the food coloring additive which industry has decreed makes them look better. After buying potato chips for a time, you begin to think they are supposed to be yellow and won't even buy them if they're not. Thus, the manufacturers who try to resist the trend risk losing business if

TABLE 10.2
Occupational Cancers

Agent	Occupation	Cancer Site
Ionizing radiations		
Radon	Certain underground miners: uranium, fluorspar, hematite	Bronchus
Xrays, radium	Radiologists, radiographers	Skin
Radium	Luminous dial painters	Bone
Ultraviolet light	Farmers, sailors	Skin
Polycyclic hydrocarbons in soot, tar, and oil	Chimney sweepers	Scrotum
	Manufacturers of coal gas	Skin
	Many other groups of exposed industrial workers	Bronchus
2–Naphthylamine	Chemical workers	Bladder
1–Naphthylamine	Rubber workers	
	Manufacturers of coal gas	
Benzidine	Chemical workers	Bladder
4–Aminobiphenyl*		
Asbestos	Asbestos workers	Bronchus
	Shipyard and insulation workers	Pleura and peritoneum

Arsenic	Sheep dip manufacturers	Skin
	Gold miners	Bronchus
	Some vineyard workers and ore smelters	
Bis(chloromethyl)ether	Makers of ion exchange resins	Bronchus
Benzene	Workers with glues, varnishes, etc.	Marrow (leukemia)
Mustard gas*	Poison gas makers	Bronchus, larynx, nasal sinuses
Vinyl chloride*	PVC manufacturers	Liver (angiosarcoma)
Chrome ores	Chromate manufacturers	Bronchus
Nickel ore	Nickel refiners	Bronchus, nasal sinuses
Isopropyl oil	Isopropylene manufacturers	Nasal sinuses
Specific agent not identified	Hardwood furniture makers	Nasal sinuses
Specific agent not identified	Leather workers	Nasal sinuses

*First suspected of causing cancer as result of animal experiments.

they don't add coloring. The only people who gain from the situation are the manufacturers of the food coloring. The rest of us have added another useless chemical to our diet, which may have long-term negative effects and which may interact with one of the other harmful chemicals in our diets to produce disease. The food is not safer; it doesn't taste better; it isn't cheaper; it doesn't last any longer.

Similar arguments can be made about occupational exposure to new chemicals. The argument we spoke of earlier was about the conflict between two notions: (1) that if a substance seems safe in short-run testing, then it should be considered safe and used at will and (2) that no substance to which the human body has never before been exposed can be considered safe in the long run—such compounds should be used only if there is no evidence that they are harmful and if substantial benefit is derived from their use by the general public. Further, if use leads to the recognition that harm does occur, then use should be stopped. The arguments in the popular press about what causes cancer and about how much federal laws impede progress fail to recognize that there are only three sources of evidence that anything causes cancer: (1) epidemiologic evidence from human populations exposed to the substance (i.e., the substance is already being used on a large scale); (2) evidence from animal studies; and (3) indirect evidence from studies of chemical structure (e.g., this chemical is similar to another one which we know causes cancer), tissue cultures (e.g., the chemical produces mutations in cells that are cultured), and other short-term studies which relate to carcinogenicity.[6] None of these sources is perfect, *but there are no others*. Special interest groups generally refuse to accept any of these as adequate. We need human studies, properly designed and controlled, they say, neglecting to mention that such studies are unethical, impossibly expensive, and require too much time to accomplish.

The controversial Delaney Amendment, which specifies that substances shown to produce cancer in any dose in laboratory animals cannot be used in food products, resulted from a recognition that the kinds of knowledge available to make these decisions were imperfect. There may be better ways to make these decisions, using guidelines which involve all three of the above sources of information, but simply abandoning the requirements of this law—which frequently is recommended—invites an increase in cancer.

Of the hundreds of thousands of chemicals to which Americans are exposed in one way or another, only some seven thousand have been subjected to long-term assays sufficient to determine their potential for carcinogenicity.[7] Of these, about one thousand have shown evidence of being cancer inducers. These tests almost never involve multiple exposure, but examine each substance individually. Human evidence of carcinogenicity exists for some twenty-six substances, only six of which were first identified in laboratory-based studies. The remainder were discovered through epidemiologic investigations. The vast majority of chemicals with laboratory evidence of mutagenicity have not been epidemiologically examined in humans.

Lester Breslow, former dean of the School of Public Health at the University of California in Los Angeles, has spent many years investigating the prevention of cancer. During a visit to Norway in 1977, Dr. Breslow was interviewed on this subject. He said:

> Environmentally induced cancer occurs mostly ten to thirty years after the exposure. As we introduce new technology in industry, new chemicals, we do not know in most cases the ultimate potential for carcinogenesis or other factors adverse to health. This does not mean that we should stop developing new technology, but we should intensify manyfold the investigations of the relationship between environmental agents and cancer. . . . I want to emphasize that all this should be done *in public*. There was a time when industry took the position that this was a matter only for the industry to be knowledgeable about. With that position the Dupont Chemical Company of

the United States managed to conceal hundreds of cases of bladder cancer among workers exposed to certain dye manufacturing processes over a period of several decades. We can no longer tolerate that kind of privacy.[8]

Once again, politics and science become enmeshed. Science cannot provide absolute answers to questions which have social, philosophical, and political ramifications. The confusion and distrust toward science result from our refusal to acknowledge the limitations of science and the responsibilities of society.

Of course, numerous other controversies surround the causes of cancer. Does a high-fat diet cause colon and breast cancers? Can mood and stress make us more susceptible to cancer? What is the role of cigarette smoking in nonrespiratory cancers? And so on. These things are certain: environment affects susceptibility to cancer; the causes of cancer are difficult to study adequately; science cannot provide more than a loose framework upon which to hang our social solutions.

SOCIAL SUPPORT SYSTEMS AND HEALTH

Ten years ago, few physicians were prepared to acknowledge a role for social and psychological factors in determining physical health. Even the majority of epidemiologists were inclined to sweep under the carpet evidence from various studies suggesting that disease rates were related to social and psychologic determinants. A great change in our understanding has taken place during the last decade. It is now accepted that personality pattern (type A or type B behavior) is related to the occurrence of heart disease. A long-term study in Alameda County, California, showed that mortality rates are related to the degree of social supports each individual has. A study of major life events and social support systems in pregnant mothers concluded that the frequency of complications at the time of delivery was related to both social support systems and stressful life events.

The presence of strong social supports seemed to provide a buffer against the disrupting and negative impact of the stressful events. Gradually, we are coming to recognize that susceptibility to disease (the size of your particular dam) is related in part to social and emotional environment. Human beings are, biologically speaking, social animals. An excessive emphasis on independence, on freedom from interdependence, may be unhealthy.

A special panel on healthy Americans was convened by the U.S. government to examine what things appear to be associated with health (as opposed to things associated with particular diseases, which is the usual approach). A section of the final report from this group examines what is known about social and psychological factors and disease[9] and says that while each individual study is inconclusive, the cumulative findings strongly suggest that social supports can accomplish the following:

1. reduce the number of complications of pregnancy for women with high life stress;
2. help prevent posthospital psychological reactions in children who have had a tonsillectomy;
3. aid recovery from surgery;
4. aid recovery from illnesses such as congestive heart failure, tuberculosis, myocardial infarctions;
5. reduce the need for steroid therapy in adult asthmatics in periods of life stress;
6. protect against clinical depression in the face of adverse events;
7. reduce psychological distress and physiological symptomatology following job loss and bereavement;
8. protect against the development of emotional problems which can be associated with aging;
9. reduce the physiological symptomatology in those working in highly stressful job environments;
10. help keep patients in needed medical treatment and promote adherence to needed medical regimens.

What are social support systems? The literature is filled with definitions. Perhaps the clearest is that of Cobb, who conceptualizes social support as information that tells a person that he or she is loved, valued, and is a part of a network of interpersonal communication and mutual obligation.[10] In other words, when you fall down someone will be there to catch you. Should we be surprised to discover that our social nature is reflected by our biologic needs?

The problem that this sort of information has created is that no one really knows what to do about it. All right, so social support systems are good things to have. Now what? Since our model of health is built on a foundation of medical care, doctors are not trained to improve social support systems, nor should they be expected to. The medical care system provides no alternative source of assistance. The physician, untrained with respect to the niceties of social and psychological needs, emphasizes immediate pathology. The patient, sick with frequent minor illnesses, goes to the doctor and receives care for each of those illnesses on an individual basis. No one is trained to observe that this pattern of frequent illness seems to reflect a generalized enhanced susceptibility to disease and to ask where this increased susceptibility originates. If the question were asked, there is no source that can render appropriate care. Nor will there be such a source until we surrender our current concepts of health and disease, our notion that each illness has a beginning and end and has a specific treatment which need be rendered only after the onset of symptoms.

Epidemiologic investigations have succeeded in establishing a conceptual relationship between psychology, emotion, and illness. Because the relationship is broad, relating to susceptibility rather than to specific disease, scientific investigations probably cannot take us much farther, at least not in a conceptual sense. The problem is that we need deep interpersonal contacts to be healthy. The solution is not a scientific one.

Chapter 11
Promoting Personal Health

When You Want Something Done Right, Do It Yourself

Take care of yourself, and be of good hope and cheer: this works a true miracle in healing.

—Petrarch

Originally I had not intended to include a chapter detailing my thoughts on how to become and remain healthy in mind and body. But, I got to telling myself that some readers might feel cheated. Having acquired this book in a search for The Answer, they would have plowed through ten challenging chapters, only to find themselves left to their own devices. (Besides, after ten years of teaching, evaluating, and researching health and medical care practices, I cannot resist inserting my own biased opinions into the subject.)

In January of 1981, the U.S. Department of Health and Human Services released a document entitled *Promoting Health, Preventing Disease. Objectives for the Nation.*[1] This document was produced after a year-long process that involved hundreds of persons in and out of government. It is designed to project health needs and goals over the next ten-year period. While I have my disagreements with this publication, it is a fine statement of problems and the beginnings of solutions. (I lean toward more radical and fundamental solutions than does the Department of Health and Human Services.) This document is used heavily in the following discussion, which is devoted to problems leading to premature death, disability, and general lack of well-being and the most feasible approaches to solving them. Medical headlines may spotlight other issues or alternative approaches, but, given current knowledge, such headlines ought to be viewed skeptically, and the tools discussed earlier for evaluating their claims should be applied to them.

Everyone has a favorite "most important health problem." The following is a review of major health problems, and no particular order of importance is intended. They are all important.

CIGARETTE SMOKING

The government report on promoting health and preventing disease calls the use of cigarettes "the single most important preventable cause of death and disease." Cigarette smoking is associated with heart and blood vessel disease (the nation's leading causes of death); cancers of the lung, larynx, pharynx, mouth, esophagus, pancreas, and bladder (the number two cause of death); chronic bronchitis and emphysema; respiratory infections; and ulcers. It produces premature wrinkling of the skin, bad breath, and is the leading cause of household fires. The combined costs of tobacco products, tobacco subsidies, illness, and fire damage each year probably exceed those of every department of the federal government except Defense and Health and Human Services.

The report *Promoting Health, Preventing Disease* makes these points about smoking:

1. Cigarette smoking is responsible for approximately 320,000 deaths annually in the United States alone.
2. Lung cancer is the leading cause of cancer deaths among men. The rise in smoking among women will make lung cancer the leading cause for females by 1983.
3. Cigarette smoking *causes* coronary heart disease, arteriosclerotic peripheral vascular disease, and all of the cancers listed above.
4. Cigarette smoking during pregnancy leads to retarded fetal growth, increased risk of abortion and prenatal death, and some impairment of growth and development during childhood.
5. Cigarette smoking acts to multiply the increased risk of illness resulting from the taking of oral contraceptives.
6. Passive inhalation of cigarette smoke can precipitate or exacerbate symptoms of asthma, heart, and respiratory diseases. Pneumonia and bronchitis are more common among children of parents who smoke.
7. Smoking causes 29 percent of fatal house fires.
8. Ten years after cessation of smoking, death rates for lung cancer and other smoking-related diseases approach those of nonsmokers.

Anyone who has ever attempted to quit a long-term smoking habit has discovered that it is not a simple matter. The addiction is powerful, both psychologically and physiologically. An individual who has smoked a pack a day for ten years has lit up more often than he or she has performed any other function in life, save breathing. Telling someone who smokes that the habit is bad is not the solution. Fundamental political and social actions must change the factors that lead to cigarette smoking in the first place. Physicians and other health practitioners must pay attention to patients' smoking, constantly reinforcing the need to quit. Smoking cessation programs must be integrated into the health care system, because not smoking is so essential to good health. Currently, tobacco companies spend $1 billion a year convincing us to smoke. The government spends millions of dollars to support tobacco growing, so that it is more profitable for the farmer to produce cigarettes than it is to grow food.

Smokers and nonsmokers alike must recognize the depth of this problem and begin to support each other in its solution. Anyone who smokes more than ten cigarettes a day, is wasting time eating right or running or engaging in any other activity for the sake of improving health.

ALCOHOL AND OTHER DRUGS

Alcohol contributed to approximately 87,000 deaths in the United States in 1975 alone. It is a contributing factor in nearly half of all fatal auto accidents and causes between 1,400 and 2,000 birth defects each year. Even small amounts of alcohol during pregnancy can produce fetal death or defect. Except during pregnancy, moderate amounts of alcohol do not appear to cause ill health and may, in fact, lead to a reduction in the risk of heart disease. People who drink heavily (and those who smoke heavily, for that matter) do so for reasons. The drinking (or smoking or drug of some other sort) fills a need. In general, our approach to treating these problems is to focus on the specific behavior rather than the underlying factors which led to it. This produces transient solutions at best. Alcoholics Anonymous works for many because it deals with the lifestyle of the alcoholic and not just the act of drinking. Until other programs deal with these underlying issues, they will not have long-term success. Long-term evaluations of alcohol and drug treatment programs have been disappointing, yet we have failed to learn from our mistakes. If it "sounds" good, we persist in our futile efforts.

Our attention to drug problems has involved addressing immediate rather than underlying causes. Prevention has failed for many of the same reasons that treatment has failed. Drugs may provide an escape from a society that provides little that is meaningful and creative for its citizens to do. The human spirit is nurtured by a sense of interdependency and creativity. We all need to be needed and to feel that we are contributing. Shape prevention and treatment programs around social changes in those directions, and they will be more successful.

NUTRITION

More is known about the nutrition of cats and dogs than about that of humans. Food preferences have always been sacrosanct, and probably that was appropriate until giant food corporations began trying to create demands for foodstuffs that, largely for cost considerations, departed further and further from the constituents of the diet on which humans evolved. And foods which had once been occasional and harmless luxuries became frequent and thus harmful parts of daily meals.

For starters, the human body did not evolve on a diet of fatty hamburgers, french fries and ice cream. Through most of mankind's existence a normal diet has consisted of raw or slightly cooked vegetables, fresh fruits, and occasional lean meat. There are, of course, exceptions to this generalization. The Masai of East Africa have eaten a high fat diet for thousands of years. But this has been coupled with a biologic mechanism for metabolizing dietary fat that is distinctive to them and also with high levels of physical activity throughout life. They also share with most other primitive peoples relatively short life expectancies because of high rates of illnesses which we are protected from by our public health programs. Thus, many of them don't live long enough to suffer from heart disease.

Too much food makes us obese, and obesity leads to hypertension and elevated levels of blood cholesterol. Too much fat in our food also raises cholesterol in the blood and almost certainly contributes to heart disease. Remember, societies that eat low-fat diets almost never have heart disease; those that eat high-fat diets *usually* have high rates.

Another problem exists with typical American high-fat, low-fiber diets that is seldom discussed in print, but to which any vegetarian or semivegetarian can attest. A high-fat meal leaves the consumer feeling full and lethargic. A low-fat diet leaves eaters far more energetic and vigorous. Try it for a week and see for yourself.

Changing our national diet is an overwhelming task. We have enormous institutions based on meeting the demands of present appetites. These demands center around high-fat, high sugar, and low-fiber tastes. It takes more than twice as many carbohydrates to produce the same number of calories in a similar amount of fat. People who think potatoes and bread are fattening don't know much about nutrition. Complex carbohydrates—starches such as potatoes, brown rice, whole-grain breads, bulgar wheat, beans—are lower in calories (unless cooked in fat or doused with butter) than meats of even the leanest variety. Food processing removes much of the value from many of our commonest foodstuffs. White bread of the kind called "balloon bread" when I was a child has many of the natural vitamins and minerals removed and has almost no fiber, an essential ingredient for proper digestion. Many such products are "enriched," but the artificially replaced vitamins and minerals are often poorly absorbed into the body and are, consequently, less useful. Whole-grain breads are more nutritious, and they taste considerably better.

"But I like balloon bread," I've heard people say. "It tastes better to me." Food tastes are learned, and it is important to recall that when trying to change your diet. Any departure from what you are used to will be strange, somehow "not quite right."

Steak lovers can learn to hate vegetables, and vegetarians can learn to hate meat. It's all a matter of practice.

Incidentally, I am not necessarily recommending vegetarianism. I am suggesting that Americans would be healthier and feel better if they ate less sugar, less fat, and more complex carbohydrates. Protein has not even entered into this conversation. Americans seem to have a fixation about protein. "Where will my protein come from?" they want to know. While protein is, indeed, essential to growth and development, protein deprivation is one of the rarest medical conditions in the United States. People who eat no meat of any kind *and* no dairy products need to be concerned about their protein sources. There are countless books to guide them in getting sufficient and appropriate proteins from their diets. For the rest of us, experiencing protein problems is considerably less likely than being struck by lightning.

Most Americans consume too much salt. Salt leads to water retention and an increase in blood pressure. Studies have shown that high salt users, if deprived of salt for a period and subsequently allowed to use as much salt as desired, will select much lower amounts than they previously used. Apparently, their "salt sensors" are somehow reset by the deprivation so that less salt becomes enough.

It is difficult to cut down on salt if you use processed foods. Canned soups, preserved meats, pickles, and packaged mixes all contain high levels of sodium and contribute to the high prevalence of hypertension.

BLOOD PRESSURE

Thirty years ago doctors paid little attention to blood pressure unless it reached such extreme levels that the affected person was in imminent danger of death. People with lower levels were free from symptoms. Epidemiologic studies, however, demonstrated that there was a direct relation over time between blood pressure and risk of dying. Later, controlled studies, in which some persons with mild high blood pressure were treated and others were not, demonstrated that standard drug treatment of hypertension resulted in significant reductions in stroke, heart disease, and other complications of high blood pressure. Sixty million Americans have elevated blood pressures and are consequently at increased risk of dying. The vast majority of these people have no symptoms and find difficulty in motivating themselves sufficiently to see a physician and take pills, which sometimes make them feel bad, to control that blood pressure. Nevertheless, the evidence is quite clear. Treatment for blood pressure saves lives. It is not a condition to be ignored.

Alternatives to drugs are available for persons with mild hypertension. Weight loss for the obese and salt-restricted diets lead to reductions in blood pressure. Even more promising is the growing evidence that the regular practice of relaxation and meditation programs can lower blood pressure. These may or may not entirely replace the need for medications, but they are worth trying, especially in view of the fact that they have beneficial effects on mental and emotional well-being as well.

PREGNANCY AND INFANT HEALTH

Babies are more likely to die during development or to be born in poor health if their mothers smoke or use alcohol or drugs during pregnancy. Adequate, well-balanced diets during pregnancy are also important. So, too, is the need to do all we can to insure that children are not born unwanted into the world. This means that health measures begin with adequate education of early adolescent children about the physiology and psychology of sex and reproduction and also with the provision of information about acceptable means of birth control *before* pregnancy occurs.

As a generalization (to which there are, of course, exceptions) teenagers do not make good mothers or fathers. They suffer, and so do their children. Parents must recognize that no matter what they desire their adolescent children are interested in sex. They may not talk about it, because communication about that topic is often taboo in the family, but they are interested. If they aren't there is something wrong. In order to behave responsibly, they must know that their interest is normal and acceptable, and they must understand what responsible behavior is. We may differ as to what we regard as acceptable sexual behavior among adolescents, but it is clear that whatever our standards are they are not instinctive. Instinct, a result of the biologic nature of mankind (and not the devil), urges people to have sex. Condemnation and the withholding of knowledge are denials of reality and major contributors to both infant and maternal morbidity and mortality.

ACCIDENTS

Wearing a seat belt is like changing your diet. If you do it for a while, you won't feel right when you don't. I have been in two accidents in which seat belts saved me from serious injury or death. Use them. Also use safety equipment provided at work for hazardous duty. Not doing so isn't brave, it's stupid. Accidents are the leading cause of death for persons between one and thirty-eight years of age. In 1978, 10,700 children below age fifteen were killed in accidents. Most were in automobiles (using seat belts would have saved more than half those lives). Fire was the next most common cause of death in children (smoking again, primarily). There were 52,400 automobile accident deaths in 1978 and two million disabling injuries. Speeding, drinking, and not using seat belts were the primary contributors. The preventive measures are partly obvious, partly not so obvious. It's simple to preach Don't speed, don't drink, and use seat belts. Those actions, taken at the individual level, will do a great deal to protect and maintain health. On a larger scale, there are complex social and legal problems involved in dealing with this important health problem.

EXERCISE

Exercise is more than a means for toning the body—it is therapy and it affects mental as well as physical well-being. I believe that sedentary living not only makes us fat, lethargic, and possessors of a poor cardiovascular system, it also contributes to irritability, depression, and other negative mood states. To be effective, exercise must be aerobic. That is, exertion should never be so heavy that the blood cannot supply the muscles as much oxygen as they are burning up. If you exercise to the point of fatigue, you are better off in an armchair. Exercise should raise the pulse rate, usually about two-fold. A general rule of thumb for healthy persons is that the pulse should not exceed 200 minus a person's age. That is, a forty-year-old man should not raise his pulse above 160 beats per minute. The amount of exercise a given person can accomplish before his or her pulse exceeds that level will increase dramatically with gradual conditioning. Finally, exercise must be regular—at least three times a week. The weekend athlete is also better off in an armchair.

Follow these three basic rules of exercise:

1. Do not exercise to the point of exhaustion.
2. Exercise hard enough to raise the pulse rate as described above.
3. Exercise in this manner at least three times a week.

If you pursue such a program, your mental and physical state of well-being will improve drastically. If you have some serious illness, especially relating to the cardiovascular system, consult with your doctor before beginning any exercise program.

STRESS, VIOLENCE,
AND WELL-BEING

At first glance it may seem that these three form a strange grouping. Since this chapter is based on opinion rather than evidence, however, I offer no apologies. Contemporary American society suffers from serious pathology. Homocide, suicide, and violent crimes are so prevalent that we think it normal to fortify our homes, carry weapons, keep loaded guns in the house, train our children to distrust strangers, and avoid interpersonal contacts with any degree of emotional intimacy except with family members. We all have our scapegoats—the rich, the poor, blacks, Jews, Chicanos, whites, corporations, politicians, tenants, landlords. It doesn't matter whose name is filled in on the blank, the effect is the same. Our inner cities often appear more like war zones than residential areas for millions of people. We know the psychological trauma that can result from actual war, but we neglect to realize that for millions of Americans growing up in a war zone is the norm. Throwing gang members into jail won't change that, and neither will more police, more burglar alarms, and more guns in the home. People who own guns have a distressing tendency to get shot with them.

Within the past ten years, the relationships between stress and health have become an acceptable subject for government funded scientific research. For decades a few intrepid scientists persisted in asking questions about the subject, despite almost universal derision from the health care community. Our state of knowledge about this field is rudimentary compared to our understanding of the relation of diet to heart disease, for example. Still, it is clear that the social support systems discussed in chapter 10 are important. For health reasons we need to know that in times of crisis there are friends and relatives around to support us, keep us from stumbling, help us realize that this is not the end. People who have been trained to distrust strangers have trouble forming intimate ties. Yet a sense of interdependence appears to be important to sustaining well-being. We need to be needed, both psychologically and physiologically. Life stresses, such as divorce, death of a spouse, and financial problems, are associated with an increased risk of physical disease, but apparently only in those persons who lack strong social support systems.

Learning to love others is not an easy task for people raised in a society that stresses suspicion and fear, and where the quickest way to get rich is through suing a neighbor. But loving is not simply a good feeling in the chest enjoyed by the sentimental. It is a social, biologic, and physiologic necessity. It sustains optimal functioning of body and mind. Unfortunately, discussing love in English is not easy. There is only one word, yet there are so many different meanings we apply to it. One of the more common deals with ownership. When we say, I love you, we often mean I own you. That is not the kind of love I am discussing here.

One of the most useful means for improving life is to permit ourselves to recognize and acknowledge the humanness of others. If certain jobs are stultifying and oppressive, it has much to do with the fact that neither employers nor employees see the humanity in each other. And it is fruitless to wait around expecting the other guy to do it first. We have a value system that justifies almost any action on the basis of profit. How often have you heard (or expressed) variations on this remark: "Well, it's too bad, but it just doesn't make financial sense not to . . ." In a society where all other values are subservient to profit, and where profit depends on somehow coming out on top of the competition, personal trust and caring are difficult, to say the least. J. Krishnamurti, an Indian sage, was once asked by a child why the anger of people who professed to love him was so intense. His reply is worth quoting here, because it so clearly explains the kind of caring we need to do for others in order to benefit ourselves:

First of all, do you love anybody? Do you know what it is to love? It is to give completely your mind, your heart, your whole being and not ask a thing in return, not put out a begging bowl to receive love. . . . And why do we get angry when we love somebody with the ordinary, so-called love? It is because we are not getting something we expect from that person, is it not? . . . You are expecting something from him, and when that expectation is not fulfilled you are disappointed—which means, that inwardly, psychologically you are depending on that person. So whenever there is psychological dependence, there must be frustration; and frustration inevitably breeds anger, bitterness, jealousy, and various other forms of conflict.[2]

Violence, purposelessness, stress, and loneliness are neither new nor unique to contemporary society. But they are unusually prevalent in the United States, and that is a result of both personal choice and social norms that facilitate bad choices. It is possible for anyone to learn to relate meaningfully to others but, like quitting smoking, it takes a great deal of conscious effort to change old patterns into new ones. It requires that we acknowledge our real feelings to ourselves and that we share those feelings with others. Learning to do this is facilitated by a sound diet, by exercise, and by daily practice of any of a number of disciplined forms of relaxation and meditation. The latter helps the mind to become more objective and less reactive, and encourages the body to relax so that attention can be focussed on a balanced center.

To summarize, do the things listed below. Numbers 1 through 6 are based on a solid, sound scientific footing that can meet the tests for acceptable data discussed throughout this book. Numbers 7, 8, and 9 are based on a less secure scientific footing, but my opinion is that they are sound and even more fundamental than the first six. Further, there is data to support 7, 8, and 9, but it is of a more preliminary nature and likely to remain so. Quantifying love and trust is difficult, so formal studies are not very satisfactory.

Here are my nine epidemiologically-derived guides to health:

1. If you smoke, quit.
2. If you use any drug (including alcohol) to the point where you need it, stop it entirely. Use no cigarettes, alcohol, or drugs during pregnancy.
3. Eat a balanced low-fat, high-fiber diet.
4. Control high blood pressure.
5. Wear seat belts.
6. Exercise regularly, but not to exhaustion.
7. Learn about your own sexuality and teach your children.
8. Meditate daily.
9. Learn to love and to trust.

Where are the debates over coffee and cancer of the pancreas? What about ginseng and camomile teas, vitamins, sedatives, and annual physical examinations? Why haven't I dealt with the problem of drinking water which is filled with chemicals or cooking with aluminum pots? Where are the advances in surgery, the importance of having strep throat treated with penicillin, the naturopathic remedies, the back manipulations, and countless other potentially useful practices? All of those things may contribute to health. The evidence as to which are more and which are less useful is not secure, but none is as important as the measures that have been discussed. If you vigorously pursue some other practice, ignoring the ones discussed, you are doing little to maintain health except giving yourself some peace of mind by rationalizing.

Chapter 12
Overview

Is the Tail Wagging the Dog?

Clearly, health cannot be dissociated from any of the factors that influence human welfare and happiness, and yet it is not the function of medicine to become identified with political action, were it only for the reason that medical training does not necessarily impart to physicians the wisdom and skill required to deal with sociopolitical problems.

—Rene Dubos

At a cost approaching $300 billion in 1981 the United States has built an almost inconceivably vast medical care complex. No other society in the history of the planet has remotely approached the scale of our mammoth health industry. Yet, we are told, national health insurance is too expensive, beyond our means. But there are a number of nations which have state-supported health care, lower medical care budgets, and better health indices. What is wrong?

It has been more than twenty years since Rene Dubos published his powerful and insightful book, *Mirage of Health*.[1] Dubos traced the historical roots of modern medicine in an effort to demonstrate how so enormous a system evolved and how it succeeded in so distorting popular notions of health and disease that even its practitioners are unaware that they have not been trained in the maintenance of health, but rather in the treatment of specific diseases. The *health care* system (as opposed to the *disease treatment* system) in the United States, and to a lesser degree in most other nations, is relatively primitive and receives only a small fraction of the resources lavished on the treatment of disease. This is not totally inappropriate, since that ounce of prevention truly is worth a pound of cure. But the imbalance is so extreme that continued efforts to reduce death and morbidity rates have led to the infusion of countless billions of dollars into medical care systems that have little hope of doing more than replacing one disease with another.

The response of the medical care system to allegations of this sort is usually to dismiss the argument out of hand or to ask for the data proving that there are effective means for preventing disease. The data are there. They do not exist in the form of laboratory experiments, but rather in the vast body of epidemiologic and sociologic studies which consistently show that certain behaviors and situations are more conducive to good mental and physical health than are others. But the medical care system is not structured to respond to those needs, nor should it necessarily be. Physicians, nurses, hospitals, and clinics have as their proper focus the care of disease. We must disabuse ourselves of the notion that caring for disease and maintaining health are the same activity. Asking a doctor about dieting or sexual problems or emotional difficulties is not unlike asking a grocer to repair an electronic calculator. Now and again you may find one who can do it, but usually the advice you receive won't make any sense at all.

Several years ago, when I worked in a family planning clinic in Oakland, California, a woman of twenty-five or so was brought into my office. She was tearful, upset, and obviously concerned about something. When I asked her what the problem was, she told me that it was painful for her to have inter-

course with her husband more than once a week. She had a
vaginal irritation and slight discharge, both symptoms of a
common and mild vaginal infection. She had gone to her own
gynecologist (who had been caring for her for seven years) with
her problem. He looked at her and uttered stonily, "Only an
animal wants it more than once a week," then sent her home
without treatment. Being underinformed (as so many people
are) about sexual matters, the woman was genuinely afraid that
she was a nymphomaniac because she and her husband liked
to make love more than once a week. While there are many
physicians who care for and understand their patients' needs,
there are too many like this one, who used his license to create
a new pathology. And there will continue to be physicians
like this as long as counseling skills, sexuality, psychology, and
sensitivity are considered to be of secondary value in medical
training.

Disease is the end result of a long process that is potentially
interruptable at many stages before the onset of symptoms. Yet
our efforts at prevention—national health insurance, health
maintenance organizations, annual physical examinations, etc.
—almost never focus on truly preventive activities. Our legisla-
tures undermine the efforts of public health agencies—the only
organized bodies of any size which do attempt to maintain
at least physical health—with laws that treat economic gain as
a higher goal than social, mental, and physical well-being.
Dubos compares modern medicine to a classic Western movie
script: a lone horseman rides into town, shoots the villains, and
rides off into the sunset while the grateful citizens wave good-
bye. The script is lovely, but what has the hero changed? The
social conditions which produced one set of villains will soon
produce another.

Health is not the only area which uses this sort of reasoning:

The Coleman Report shocked the academic world with data
strongly suggesting that a child's academic achievement de-

pended primarily on the home environment, not the school. Every group of distinguished citizens ever asked to be on a crime commission has come solidly to the conclusion that no amount of policy, judges, courts, or laws will alter crime rates if the environment of poverty persists. Health should be added to this list. Education, crime, and health make an imposing array. We can continue the patchwork approach, hoping that our "system" will not need much alteration. We can exist with the lazy wish that more police will stop crime, more school buildings and teachers will make our children smarter, and more hospitals and doctors will make our society healthy. Or we can approach these problems in terms of primary prevention.[2]

MAKING PERSONAL HEALTH DECISIONS

In some respects, human beings are quite like biological computers. Practiced behavior becomes automatic so that it can be performed without thinking. The best right-handed tennis player in the world will look clumsy if he tries to play left handed. With practice, it is possible to learn to perform actions with our reluctant opposite hand, but it takes time. Intellectual knowledge of how to carry out an action is only a small first step. Practice is what makes it part of us.

We have been raised in a society in which junk foods are treated as rewards, cigarette smoking is portrayed as sensuous and sexually attractive, competitiveness and upward mobility are highly valued, and disease care is called health care. The fact that these are all ingrained actions and ideas makes it that much more difficult to change them. But if we would be happy and well in this life we must do some changing, both on a personal and societal level. Here are some suggestions to be repeated like mantras:

1. It is possible to be healthier and happier than I am, no matter how good or how bad I feel at the present time.

2. Ways to achieve better health are known and they are generally not complex.
3. Changes are best achieved by carefully choosing one or two small, desired alterations and committing myself to them.
4. The changes that are best for me to make can be determined only by sitting quietly and listening to my inner voice. If I don't feel deeply motivated, I will not succeed.
5. I will largely ignore scientific health information in the popular press unless it appears consistently and is widely accepted.
6. Success is more likely if I pick clear and achievable goals, and proceed slowly toward them.
7. Success will be certain only when changes are practiced to the point that they become automatic.
8. Few meaningful answers lie outside myself.

THE MEDICAL MODEL

In 1977 George Engel published an article calling for a change in our basic notions of health and disease.[3] He pointed out that the dominant model of disease in current use assumes that illness is "fully accounted for by deviations from the norm of measurable biological (somatic) variables," leaving no place for social, psychologic, and behavioral dimensions of ill health, and using only physical tools to study biological systems. In our culture, he points out:

> the attitudes and belief systems of physicians are molded by this model long before they embark on their professional education, which in turn reinforces it without necessarily clarifying how its use for social adaptation contrasts with its use for scientific research. The biomedical model has thus become a cultural imperative, its limitations easily overlooked. In brief, it has now acquired the status of *dogma*. In science, a model is revised or abandoned when it fails to account adequately for all the data.

A dogma, on the other hand, requires that discrepant data be forced to fit the model or be excluded.[4]

Scientists are always in danger of lapsing into dogma. From the inquisition of Galileo to the modern day ostracization of Pauling and Szent-Gorgy for their unorthodox theories, the ranks of establishment scientists have included a fair number of dogmatists.

Engel proposes what he terms a "biopsychosocial" model of health. This model includes the patient as a person rather than simply his or her laboratory readings and physical findings. In current health systems, there is no response to disease (i.e., not "feeling right"), but only to demonstrable biologic abnormality. The fact that no abnormality is detected may indicate that diagnostic efforts have been inadequate, that the symptoms are not being physically manifested, or that the results of the tests have been improperly interpreted. It never means that the patient who feels bad is, in fact, well. Wellness, after all, is ultimately a subjective matter. The biopsychosocial model would:

> acknowledge the fundamental fact that the patient comes to the physician because either he does not know what is wrong, or if he does, he feels incapable of helping himself. The psychobiological unity of man requires that the physician accept the responsibility to evaluate whatever problems the patient presents and recommend a course of action, including referral to other helping professions. Hence the physician's basic professional knowledge and skills must span the social, psychological, and biological, for his decisions and actions on the patient's behalf involve all three.[5]

This notion also implies that some responsibility for health be shared by each individual. Industries have frequently seized on this quite reasonable idea to justify all manner of outrageous activities, from the marketing of adulterated, non-nutritious snack foods to the pollution of rivers and oceans, claiming that public health is an individual responsibility and not really their affair. And while health is everybody's business, every individual ought to do all the things that are within his or her power to undertake. In themselves, these measures (discussed in chapter 11) may not be enough to assure marvelous health, but without them, it is useless to expect a doctor or society to protect personal health.

Good health is thoroughly intertwined with mental and social well-being. Although there is a side of each of us—usually lurking slightly below the conscious level—that wishes to be taken care of, coddled, and permitted excesses without the necessity of paying penalties, that side is as purely wishful as a trip to Oz with Dorothy and Toto. We cannot feel optimally well, either physically or emotionally, unless we come to grips with this tendency to pass the buck. It isn't fair to ourselves or the doctor, chiropractor, naturopath, or public health department. As human beings we are capable of excellence. In a sense, it is our destiny to do the best we can at everything we attempt, not to be better than anyone else, not to be perfect, but simply to do our best. When we tolerate what our inner selves tell us is less than our best, we are making ourselves a little less human, a little less conscious, and a little less healthy.

Use the guidelines provided in this book to assist in decision making about health priorities. There is no balance in the popular press, only stories which reflect today's most "hype-able" events. Provide your own balance.

The techniques for decision-making discussed here can be applied to other areas besides health. The rational and the nonrational worlds, the scientific and the emotional-mental-mystical, do not conflict; they complement one another. Health and well-being require their integration.

Notes

1/What Epidemiology Is

1. David E. Lilienfeld, "Definitions of Epidemiology," *American Journal of Epidemiology* 107 (1978): 87–90.
2. Berton Roueche, *Annals of Epidemiology* (Boston: Little, Brown, 1967).
3. John G. Fuller, *Fever!* (New York: Reader's Digest Press, 1974).
4. Geoffrey Rose and D. J. P. Barker, "Epidemiology for the Uninitiated: What Is Epidemiology?" *British Medical Journal* 2 (1978): 803–4.
5. John Ryle, *Changing Disciplines* (London: Oxford University Press, 1948).
6. John N. Morris, *The Uses of Epidemiology* (Edinburgh: E. and S. Livingston, 1964).

2/A Brief History of the Field

1. Hippocrates, *On Airs, Waters and Places,* translated and published in *Medical Classics* 3(1938): 19–42.
2. John Graunt, *Natural and Political Observations Made upon the Bills of Mortality,* London, 1662 (Baltimore: Johns Hopkins University Press, 1939).
3. James Lind, *A Treatise of the Scurvy,* Edinburgh, 1753, in C. P.

Steward and D. Guthrie, eds., *Lind's Treatise on Scurvy* (Edinburgh: University Press, 1953).

4. George Baker, *An Essay Concerning the Cause of the Endemial Colic of Devonshire*, London, 1768 (New York: Delta Omega Society, 1958).

5. James Earle, *The Original Works of Percival Pott*, F.R.S., Vol. 3, Cancer Scroti (London: J. Johnson, 1763).

6. Peter L. Panum, "Observations Made during the Epidemic of Measles on the Faroe Islands in the Year 1846," in *Panum on Measles* (New York: APHA, Delta Omega Society, 1940).

7. John Snow, *On the Mode of Communication of Cholera*, 2nd ed., London, 1855, in *Snow on Cholera*, (New York: Commonwealth Fund, 1936; reprint, New York: Hafner, 1965).

8. Henry Whitehead, *Experience of a London Curate* (London: Clapham, 1874).

9. Bernard Barber, "Resistance by Scientists to Scientific Discovery," *Science* 134 (1961): 596–602.

3/Populations and Peoples

1. Kenneth J. Rothman, "The Rise and Fall of Epidemiology, 1950–2000 A.D.," *New England Journal of Medicine* 304 (1981): 600–602.

2. Milton Terris, "Epidemiology as a Guide to Health Policy," *Annual Review of Public Health* 1(1980): 323–44.

4/The Transmission and Prevention of Illness

1. Abram S. Berenson, *Control of Communicable Diseases in Man*, 12th ed. (Washington, D.C.: American Public Health Association, 1975).

2. Institute of Medicine, National Academy of Sciences, *Healthy People. The Surgeon General's Report on Health Promotion and Disease Prevention*, Background Papers, 1979, U.S. Depart-

ment of Health, Education, and Welfare, Public Health Service, DHEW Publication No. (PHS) 79-55071A (Washington, D.C.: Government Printing Office, 1979).

5/Finding the Causes

1. W. W. May, "The Composition and Function of Ethical Committees," *Journal of Medical Ethics* 1(1975): 23–29.
2. Paavo Airola, *Are You Confused?* (Phoenix, Ariz.: Health Plus Pub., 1971).
3. Douglas B. Altman, "Statistics and Ethics in Medical Research: Collecting and Screening Data," *British Medical Journal* 281 (1980): 1399–1401.

6/Statistics and the Misuse of Information

1. William B. Kannel, "Some Lessons in Cardiovascular Epidemiology from Framingham," *American Journal of Cardiology* 37 (1976): 269–82.

7/Screening for Disease

1. J. M. G. Wilson and G. Jungner, *Principles and Practices of Screening for Disease* (Geneva: World Health Organization, 1968). Reprinted with the permission of the publisher.
2. Jean L. Marx, "The Annual Pap Smear: An Idea Whose Time Has Gone?" *Science* 205(1979): 177–78.
3. E. George Knox, "The Evaluation of Mass Screening Programmes for Cervical Cancer," *Tumori* 62(1976): 111–42.
4. Loring G. Dales, Gary D. Friedman, and Morris F. Collen, "Evaluation of a Periodic Multiphasic Health Checkup," *Methods of Information in Medicine* 13(1974): 140–46; Morris F.

Collen, *Multiphasic Health Testing Services*, MHTS (New York: John Wiley, 1972).

5. Claire Bombardier, Jacqueline McClaran, and David L. Sackett, "Periodic Health Examinations and Multiphasic Screening," *Canadian Medical Association Journal* 109(1973): 1123–27.

6. Thomas M. Vogt, "Risk Assessment and Health Hazard Appraisal," *Annual Review of Public Health* 2(1981): 31–47.

8/Evaluating Medical Practice

1. Edward C. Lambert, *Modern Medical Mistakes* (Bloomington: Indiana University Press, 1978).

2. "The Coronary Drug Project Research Group: Clofibrate and Niacin in Coronary Heart Disease," *Journal of the American Medical Association* 231(1975): 360–81.

3. Committee of Principal Investigators, "A Co-operative Trial in the Primary Prevention of Ischemic Heart Disease Using Clofibrate," *British Heart Journal* 40(1978): 1069–1118.

4. Bernard Lown, A. M. Fakhro, W. B. Hood, et al., "The Coronary Care Unit: New Perspectives and Directions," *Journal of the American Medical Association* 199(1967): 188–98.

5. H. G. Mather, N. G. Pearson, K. L. Q. Read, et al., "Acute Myocardial Infarction: Home and Hospital Treatment," *British Medical Journal* 7(1971): 334–38.

6. J. D. Hill, J. R. Hampton, and J. P. A. Mitchell, "A Randomized Trial of Home-Versus-Hospital Management for Patients with Suspected Myocardial Infarction," *Lancet* 1(1978): 837–41.

7. Leon Gordis, Naggan Lechaim, and James Tonascia, "Pitfalls in Evaluating the Impact of Coronary Care Units on Mortality from Myocardial Infarctions," *Johns Hopkins Medical Journal* 141(1977): 287–95.

8. John D. Bunker, Klim McPherson, and Phillip L. Henneman, "Elective Hysterectomy," in John D. Bunker, Benjamin D. Barnes, and Frederick F. Mosteller, eds., *Costs, Risks, and Benefits of Surgery* (New York: Oxford University Press, 1977).

9/Medical Care and the Public Health

1. Marc Lalonde, A *New Perspective on the Health of Canadians: A Working Document* (Ottawa: Ministry of National Health and Welfare, 1974).
2. Ibid, p. 13.
3. Archibald L. Cochrane, A. S. St. Leger, and F. Moore, "Health Service 'Input' and Mortality 'Output' in Developed Countries," *Journal of Epidemiology and Community Health* 32(1978): 200–205.

10/Some Current Controversies

1. George V. Mann, "Diet-Heart: End of an Era," *New England Journal of Medicine* 297(1977): 644–50.
2. "Diet-Heart Era: Premature Obituary?" *New England Journal of Medicine* 298(1978): 106–10.
3. John S. Garrow, "Weight penalties," *British Medical Journal* II (1979): 1171–72.
4. Richard C. LaBarba, "Experiential and Environmental Factors in Cancer: A Review of Research with Animals," *Psychosomatic Medicine* 32 (1970): 259–75.
5. Richard Doll, "Epidemiology of Cancer: Current Perspectives," *American Journal Epidemiology* 104 (1976): 396–407.
6. Interagency Regulatory Liaison Group, "Scientific Bases for Identification of Potential Carcinogens and Estimation of Risks," *Annual Review of Public Health* 1(1980): 345–93.
7. Ibid.
8. "Is There Ground for Optimism in Cancer Prevention?" *Nordisk Medicin* 92(1977): 269–71.
9. B. A. Hamburg and M. Killilea, "Relation of Social Support, Stress, Illness, and Use of Health Services," in Institute of Medicine, National Academy of Sciences, *Healthy People: The Surgeon General's Report on Health Promotion and Disease Pre-*

vention, Background Papers, 1979, U.S. Department of Health, Education, and Welfare, Public Health Service, DHEW Publication No. (PHS) 79-55071A (Washington, D.C.: Government Printing Office, 1979).

10. Sidney Cobb, "Social Support as a Moderator of Life Stress," *Psychosomatic Medicine* 38(1976): 300–314.

11/Promoting Personal Health

1. U.S., Department of Health and Human Services, *Promoting Health, Preventing Disease. Objectives for the Nation* (Washington, D.C.: Government Printing Office, 1980).

2. J. Krishnamurti, *Think on These Things* (New York: Harper and Row, 1964).

12/Overview

1. Rene Dubos, *Mirage of Health* (New York: Doubleday, 1959).

2. P. Isacson, "Poverty and Health: There's Only So Much a Doctor Can Do," *New Republic*, Dec. 14, 1974.

3. G. Engle, "The Need for a New Medical Model: A Challenge for Biomedicine," *Science* 69(1977): 129–36.

4. Ibid.

5. Ibid.

Suggested Reading

Ahmed, P. I., ed. *Toward a New Definition of Health: Psychosocial Dimensions*. New York: Plenum Press, 1979. A collection of papers on the need to redefine the traditional concept of health as the absence of disease.

Albrecht, G., and Higgins, P. G. *Health, Illness, and Medicine: A Reader in Medical Sociology*. Chicago: Rand-McNally College Pub. Co., 1979. A collection of papers providing broad insights on health, illness, and medical care.

Cameron, W. B. "The Elements of Statistical Confusion, or—What Does the Mean Mean?" *Bulletin of American Association of University Professors* 43 (1957): 33–39. A short look at the ways in which statistics can mislead, and how to be on your guard against being taken in.

Dubos, Rene. *Mirage of Health. Utopias, Progress, and Biological Change*. New York: Doubleday, 1959. A profound classic synthesis of health, disease, and the human process.

Hill, Austin Bradford. *Principles of Medical Statistics*, 9th ed. New York: Oxford University Press, 1971. Pp. 274–308. Hill's text has been reprinted many times because it is so readable, clear, and thorough. Unlike most statistical texts, it is actually fun to read.

Illich, Ivan. *Medical Nemesis: The Expropriation of Health.* Toronto: Bantam Books, 1976. A blistering attack on the medical care system. The many quotes out of context and obvious bias of the author should not obscure the meaningful points he makes. If the writing had been more tempered, this work might have had a greater impact.

Insel, Paul M., and Moos, Rudolf H. *Health and the Social Environment.* Lexington, Mass.: D. C. Heath, 1974. A collection of papers relating the social environment to health and illness.

Institute of Medicine, National Academy of Sciences. *Healthy People. The Surgeon General's Report on Health Promotion and Disease Prevention. Background Papers 1979.* U.S., Department of Health, Education, and Welfare, Public Health Service, DHEW Publication No. (PHS) 79-55071A. Washington, D.C.: Government Printing Office, 1979. A detailed review of the results of scientific studies relating human practices and behavior to health. Tends to be conservative and relies on research findings only. The results may be surprising to many.

Knox, E. George, ed. *Epidemiology in Health Care Planning. A Guide to the Uses of a Scientific Method.* New York: Oxford University Press, 1979. Illustrates how epidemiology can introduce a rational basis into planning health services and setting priorities for scarce health-care resources.

Ludwig, Edward G., and Collette, John C. "Some Misuses of Health Statistics." *Journal of the American Medical Association* 216 (1971): 493–99. Short article with marvelous examples of how to mislead a reader. Enjoyable and excellent.

Pelletier, Kenneth R. *Holistic Medicine: From Stress to Optimum Health.* New York: Delacorte, 1974. An overview of the holistic health movement from a scientific perspective.

Index